Anne Diamond

Anne Diamond has been a household name for the past 25 years, working in daily TV, radio and national newspapers. Far from being just a journalist, she pioneered breakfast TV in the early 1980s, anchoring *TVam* and interviewing global leaders, celebrities and top politicians in locations as varied as Sydney Harbour during the Australian Bicentennial, the Brandenburg Gate during the fall of the Berlin Wall, and Hollywood. She started daytime TV with the BBC, and now regularly hosts breakfast and morning radio programmes, often starting her day in the middle of the night! She is the author of many books, both fact and fiction, and is a busy mum of four boys.

Professionally, she is most proud of her reputation as a health campaigner within her TV and radio work, spearheading awareness drives on a national level concerning cervical cancer screening, autism, dyslexia and vaccination programmes. She marks as her greatest achievement the instigation and presentation of the 1991 'Back to Sleep' campaign to prevent cot death, which dramatically reduced the rate of SIDS (Sudden Infant Death Syndrome) in Britain – from around 2500 annual deaths to 300. This followed the cot death of her own son, Sebastian. For her part in saving what's estimated to be around 20,000 lives, Anne was recently awarded the College Medal of the Royal College of Paediatrics and Child Health, the only non-medic ever to receive this accolade.

Now she has turned her attention to the obesity epidemic, following her own well-publicised battle with her weight. Two years ago, Anne underwent gastric surgery – first abroad, then subsequently here in Britain. Her colourful experience has become both a warning siren and a ray of hope for many patients whose health is in danger because of their weight.

During her recent 'Get Your Life Back' tour, Anne was moved by the distress of many obese people who cannot afford or cannot face surgery, and who see no end to their plight. Some have told her that they feel suicidal over their weight, others that their life is made miserable by a condition that society says is their own fault. So how can they be treated? Who in the world knows how to help? Anne has travelled the globe, trying to find out the answers to those questions – and more.

Now she runs a free weight-loss support website, which has thousands of members and is recommended to patients by top bariatric surgeons and obesity specialists – it's called BuddyPower (www.buddypower.net) and is helping ordinary men and women to lose weight by offering them practical and emotional support, easy access to expert advice, and a blame-free environment where people can learn a new, healthy lifestyle with the help of a unique buddying system – Buddy Power! For support and further information about the issues discussed in this book visit **www.buddypower.net**

"FAT IS NOT YOUR FAULT... BUT IT IS YOUR PROBLEM"

WINNING THE FAT WAR

EXPERT WAYS TO LOSE WEIGHT IN A FAT WORLD
ANNE DIAMOND

CAPSTONE

*

CONTENTS

*

FOREWORD

*

Picasso once wrote a play in which there were two memorable characters called Thin Anxiety and Fat Anxiety. The first had been stressed to skin and bone; the second had been driven to comfort eating. The first was adrenalising so much that appetite was suppressed and the flesh fell off; the second reacted to tension by seeking a primeval calming device. As any mother knows, the best way to calm a baby is to put it to the breast, where it finds a sweet-tasting reward. The anxious adult does the next best thing by seeking sweet nourishment of other kinds – cakes, biscuits, chocolates, candies, ice creams and all the rest.

For previous generations, moments of tension were relieved by a different kind of oral comfort. As a writer, if I was stuck for a word, I would reach for a cigarette. A few puffs and the missing word would come. I had not added to my weight, but I had clogged up my lungs. Nowadays I reach instead for a peppermint and my lungs are fine, but my waistline is not. If I lived a natural lifestyle, I would not have a problem. By 'natural' I mean physically active. The human species did not evolve sitting at a desk like me. For a million years our ancestors endured the hard physical life of hunter-gatherers, and it helped to shape their bodies. Their slim figures were a testimony to their athletic way of life. Today typical city dwellers sit on their way to work, sit behind a desk in the office, then go home to sit at a computer or in front of a television set in the evening. Athletes they are not. What is amazing today is not that some people are fat, but that, given their sedentary lifestyle, many are still slim.

So the rule is simple. If you want to get fat, sit a lot and worry a lot. If you are not worried enough, just put on the television news and it will soon have you reaching for that extra chocolate biscuit.

When I made a study of people who had lived to be 100, I found that nearly all of them had enjoyed a physically strenuous life. They loved things like walking, gardening or cycling. Madame Jeanne Calment, the oldest person ever to have lived, was still riding her bicycle at the age of 100. And, although she continued to enjoy her rich French stews and cheap red wine in the years that followed, she was still as thin as a rake at 120.

There is so much talk about diet regimes these days, as though these will answer the obesity crisis that faces society, but the problem is much more basic than that, and Anne Diamond's book is an investigation into an important social issue. Anne herself is one of those lively, cheerful, warm-hearted people who, despite some well-publicised ups and downs, remains a life-enhancer for all those who know her, and it gives me great pleasure to welcome you to her common-sense treatment of an increasingly serious problem. Now read on...

Desmond Morris
Oxford, 2008

INTRODUCTION

*

T his is painful. Just sitting here typing on my computer, thinking out an introduction to this book is really, really painful. I've got such a lot to say about winning the fat war – and it needs to be said by someone brave enough to take the inevitable flak for it.

But I keep looking for something else to do instead. You know? I keep putting it off. I go downstairs for a cup of coffee. I decide it's time to clear out my email inbox. I go through my desktop deleting all the silly little video games 'shortcuts' and codecs and stuff that my kids have downloaded on to my computer when they swore blind they were doing their homework. I tidy up. I go downstairs and do the ironing, cook a meal, collect the kids from school when they could quite easily catch a bus... Anything but the pain of what I must talk about now.

Because it is about one of the most horrible episodes of my life and yet, looking back, it seems almost trivial. What sort of person gets all worked up and upset about something as unimportant their weight – about being fat? Me, that's who. And thousands like me.

Weight – obesity (how I hate that word – no matter how you try to say it, it sounds like an insult) drags you down so much heavier than mere gravity. It preys on your mind. It makes you feel so worthless, so stupid. Your brain tells you it's not such a problem.

But when you look in the mirror, your heart screams that you're a big fat slob. And then you register the pain.

Because fat matters – in oh, so many ways. And those who tell you it's silly to obsess about it are the same ones who pillory you if you start to wobble around the waist. They're the tyrants who, until now, have been allowed to dominate the media and the dieting and health industry. They're the so-called slimming and fitness experts who think it's cool to throw cream cakes at desperate fatties or yell obscenities at sweating kids in fat camps. Well, their days are over. Their nastiness, which was a novelty once upon a time, is now boring and ineffective. It's time for a little constructive compassion.

Even the Tories – whose leader, David Cameron, so recently made a posturing speech about being 'fed up hearing about those who are at risk of being fat' and promised a new, tougher stance on obesity – know that a change of direction is needed. But when I asked their health spokesman, Andrew Lansley, he modified their macho public statements significantly. He famously said there were 'no excuses for being obese'.

'I didn't mean that the state shouldn't take responsibility too,' he backtracked. 'Beating obesity is about both personal and state responsibility. But once help has been given, there are no excuses.' With that attitude, nothing is going to change. In fact, things might well get worse if left to such political insensitivity.

Only the 'swarm effect' will make a difference now. That's the new buzzword being used by the non-government organisations, the health charities, the pressure groups. Each of them is trying, in its own way, to create a better environment, a greater awareness, a better understanding. From above, it looks like chaos, a mess of initiatives – but together, that 'swarm' will have an effect – it will be felt. Good thing too.

I feel passionate about this because I have been there. I've been yelled at, I have been pelted with cruel headlines and malicious, ignorant, stinging words, and it was hell. It forced me to find another way – a better way. But it's been a long journey. I have come out the other side of that cavernous hell-hole, proud of my achievements and feeling slimmer and fitter than ever – but most of all, more easy with myself, and more caring about others who are suffering the same sort of media-inspired, frenzied-mob abuse.

'I hate being hated because I am fat,' wrote one young woman to me. 'You can see it in their eyes. It's not even pity – it's actual hatred. Yet they don't even know me!'

'The thought of a family holiday is making me so depressed, and yet I should be elated,' wrote another last summer. 'The thought of baggy T-shirts and stretch leggings, and hiding in a corner ashamed because I know people will stare and whisper...'

Did it ever occur to the critics and the fun-pokers that the vast majority of fat people actually hate being fat? That it gnaws at them until life becomes almost unbearable? I know because I have met them and I receive letters from hundreds every week. Many remember me as the skinny young thing on breakfast television in the 1980s, and the slightly more rounded mother of four on morning TV in the '90s. They say, 'If it could happen to you, it could happen to anyone!' And that makes them feel less alone.

Fat happens

It's true: fat really can happen to anyone. I tell that to the cocky young broadcasters who interview me nowadays about obesity. If they get too patronising (as so many do on this subject), I remind them that once upon a time, my bum on the TV sofa was half the size of theirs. That wipes the smirk off their faces.

One of my sons came running through to the kitchen the other day calling, 'Mum, come and see this on the computer – it's you interviewing Kylie when you were both *so young*!'

He'd been surfing through the website YouTube and had stumbled across a video clip from 1987, when I was broadcasting *Good Morning Britain* from Sydney, Australia, during the TV technicians' strike. There I was, all young and effortlessly slim, with padded shoulders and big, dangly earrings, and there was Kylie with ringletted hair and a really strong Aussie accent. She was talking about how she would like to leave *Neighbours* and try a career as a singer – just to see how it would turn out.

Then I noticed the headline accompanying the clip: it said, 'Veteran broadcaster Anne Diamond in the first big interview with Kylie'. (You know you've been in the business a few years when you're described as a veteran!) Then, and you will know how this works if you have ever surfed through YouTube, I clicked on the words 'Veteran broadcaster Anne Diamond' and up came dozens and dozens more clips. Here I was interviewing Margaret Thatcher, Dudley Moore, Nelson Mandela, Emu and even Kermit the Frog, and there I was doing aerobics in a slimming and fitness video, appearing on *Celebrity Big Brother, Stars in Your Eyes* and *Celebrity Fit Club*. And then the headlines grew a little different and rather more judgemental: 'Anne Diamond looking huge as she leaves the Big Brother house'; 'Anne Diamond turns Big Brother into Big Blubber'; and even more hurtful, 'Whatever happened to the elfin queen of breakfast television?' 'Has Anne Diamond lost her sparkle?'

Well, you certainly need a thick hide to withstand that sort of attack, don't you? I know that anyone well known has to learn to take all that sort of stuff in their stride. But it certainly taught me a thing or two about society's attitude towards obesity.

Compared with other celebrities and household names, who were caught snorting coke, visiting massage parlours and having affairs with John Major, I had committed the sin of all sins: I had put on weight. And, as Britney Spears has found out, to the media, that's worse than losing custody of your kids or being arrested and driven off in an ambulance.

Believe me, it's hard enough to lose weight once you've put it on without society throwing brickbats at you and beating you down with your own failed efforts.

It ain't rocket science...

I am so fed up with self-righteous men and women telling me that 'Losing weight isn't rocket science, you know. All you have to do is eat less and exercise more.' Because that sort of advice has landed us with an obesity epidemic. It simply has not worked, and has prevented a more constructive attitude emerging – one that might have helped long ago.

It's not that it's incorrect advice. Of course it's right. We all know that energy in must equal energy out, but that is not helpful enough. Not nowadays. Not in a world where we all live more sedentary lifestyles and are encouraged, bribed and brainwashed into eating more food, and some of it absolute junk.

There's no doubt in my mind: the media has played a culpable role in causing this epidemic too. Advertising has brainwashed us over the years to think of commercialised, branded junk food as a highly desirable luxury, as a treat we all deserve – and it is sold with all the sexualised, celebrity-endorsed razzamatazz that they use to sell cars and holidays. Then there's the unforgivable ignorance of the news media, which reports obesity stories with the blood-baying fury of salivating hyenas, eager to rip the guts out of the poor, pathetic victim. (I can just about forgive the news presenter who told me I was fat because I clearly ate too many chips and probably dipped them in mayonnaise!) Programme producers purport to treat the subject responsibly by inventing reality shows, such as *Celebrity Fit Club*, or *Too Big to Walk*, where a TV crew followed a team of hugely obese people on what seemed to me to be a foolishly long walk up and down mountains, and then allowed viewers to wallow in their distress.

Until society evolves a more compassionate attitude towards those who are already suffering from obesity, we'll never get ahead of the problem. Not only will our children suffer (and one in five is already obese here in the UK – we have the fattest kids in Europe), but we will be cruelly writing off a whole generation of mums and dads who deserve a fighting chance to reclaim their lives too.

Fat prejudice is all around us

Unlike alcoholics, drug addicts, gamblers, shopaholics or even sex offenders, the human being suffering from food addiction advertises his or her problem to the world. One of my own children pointed it out the other day. We were in the car, in a traffic jam, and my son was staring out of the window...

'Wow! Look at that enormous woman! Look, look! How on earth did she get *that fat*?'

We all looked. Sure enough, there was an absolutely huge woman wobbling past. She really was obese, in the extreme sense, if you know what I mean. Her weight must have been almost literally off the scales. She looked as though she was struggling just to walk.

'I don't understand it,' sighed another of my sons. 'How do you get that big without noticing it piling on? Surely you'd stop before you got that huge?'

It *is* hard to understand. My boys weren't meaning to be unkind – and they were asking a very important question. *The* question, in fact. And to date, I haven't found anyone who really has the answer, although some experts are at least trying to find it.

'Don't be unkind,' I told my boys. 'That woman might be dying inside. She probably hates being so fat. She might cry herself to sleep about it every night, and wake up hating herself. Please, please don't imagine that she is that way because she wants to be.'

It's totally unacceptable, cruel and ignorant to poke fun at or even point out someone who's clearly a sufferer from other diseases or disabilities. But the fatty still gets the stocks.

OK, some fat people might, just *might,* be fat and happy about it. But I know if I invented a magic slimming pill that would turn fatties into slimmies overnight, *everyone would take it.*

'I have always been fat,' wrote one member of my weight-loss support website, buddypower.net. 'My mum says she had to prick extra holes in my bottle as a baby as my face would turn blue with the effort of trying to get the milk out. I was put on my first diet aged eight – a vile Complan meal replacement thing – torture. I grew into a fat child, then a fat teenager, followed by being a fat 20-something and I'm now a fat 30-something. I have tried every diet imaginable, but am still around 6 stone overweight.

'I am generally contented, I have a very happy, loving and supportive relationship, two great kids, a job I love and plenty of good friends. I'm just not happy with *me.* I was diagnosed with type 2 diabetes in February and have struggled to reduce my blood glucose levels with diet and medication. I know I need to lose weight for the sake of my health and for my children. My husband loves me but I know he's terribly worried for me and dare not mention my weight in case it upsets me more.'

She's desperate for help. She's not daft, but she can't do it on her own – and if you've ever been there, you'll understand that.

I have been there

Oh yes, I have been there, done that, got the extra large T-shirt and even made the video. I have done every diet in the land – and put on yet more weight at the end of them. Once it loads on, it's hell's own game getting rid of it.

After the horrible headlines that followed my appearance on *Celebrity Big Brother*, I immediately starved myself and exercised like a mad thing. I lost so much weight so quickly that everyone told me I should make a fitness and slimming video. So I did. But to celebrate its release, the publishers took me to a slap-up lunch, and I never looked back. On came the weight again. And again, and again, after every diet and every gym subscription. All the weight again – and then more.

When I got to 15 stone 10 lb I was scared. I knew that just around the corner lay diabetes and the increased risk of cancer, heart disease, stroke and a shortened lifespan. You know it. That's when a little bit inside you dies. That's when you stop venturing out as much as you used to. That's when you don't go swimming with the kids because the only swimsuit that fits you looks like something meteorologists use to make weather balloons. So you just watch them from the poolside. It's when you wake up most mornings dreading having to get dressed into clothes you hate, and you go to bed every night feeling a failure because you ate a Malteser.

That's when I a friend of mine told me of someone she knew who'd had a gastric band fitted and had since lost masses of weight. Until then, I'd thought weight-loss surgery was something that only weird Americans and Sharon Osbourne went in for.

So started my colourful history with weight-loss surgery. To cut a long story short, I went to Belgium to have it done because I thought it would be cheaper and they boasted no MRSA in their hospitals. Unfortunately, they put the band in the wrong place – around the bottom of my oesophagus instead of around my stomach. No wonder it didn't work.

It was a horrible time – made even worse when my surgery became public knowledge. I got flak from all directions, not least the people on *Celebrity Fit Club*, who accused me of cheating, even though I wasn't losing weight. Hearteningly, though, I got thousands and thousands of letters from fellow sufferers who just wanted to stay in touch – too many to be able to reply personally to each – so I set up a weight-loss support website that, more than anything, relies on the power of friendship to get people through. It's called buddypower.net. Remember it – you might need it because it's one of the few places on Earth where overweight or fat or obese (whatever your word of choice) people will be treated with respect and constructive help.

Fat matters, you see. It matters to everyone. It's a matter of vanity, natural good looks and vital self-esteem. And it's also a matter of health. It is not, however, a matter of blame. Every 'real' expert I have met – and by that I mean clinicians, surgeons and scientists working at the front line of the Fat War, not self-righteous, self-styled slimming gurus on TV – is adamant that fat is no one's fault. It is marching, epidemic-like, across the globe like an unstoppable virus or plague. It is affecting almost a quarter of us who live the Western lifestyle. But it's the lifestyle that's at fault – not us personally. Until we understand that, and treat fatties with compassion and realistic help, we won't get our bodies back.

In my quest to find out how to win the fat war, I have travelled from London to New York, Sydney to San Francisco, and interviewed obesity specialists from Brazil to New Delhi, and I've come right back home, where our very own scientists are doing some of the best work on the planet. They say losing weight is damned hard – they feel they're 'having to teach patients to swim against the tide'. But there are ways to do it, and I have gleaned their top tips and ideas for you here in this book so that you can be briefed by people who are real experts in the field, not those who think bullying is the answer.

Buddying, not bullying – that's the motto I've adopted for my BuddyPower website. I hope it will benefit all of us.

*

MY STORY

*

Obesity surgery is a treatment in its relative infancy. They have been at it, in any great numbers, for only about 20 years. But from the experience now of thousands, we can be confident that it *is* an effective treatment for many, many patients. Some lose all their excess weight, others lose a significant proportion of it. For nearly everyone, it improves the quality of their life and their health.

I'm not advocating surgery for all. In fact, I'm not advocating it for anyone. It is entirely a personal choice, and a very private one too. I can only tell you my experiences and give you as much information as I can so that you are better informed than I was when I first felt desperate enough to do it.

I hate that word 'desperate'. The papers love to use it about any fattie who dreams of a slimmer body. It implies a touch of sadness, and madness. It's been used so many times to describe me!

You don't have to be sad or mad to be desperate about your weight and determined to do something about it. In fact, I reckon it takes courage because it is about facing up to your demon, and deciding to take the ultimate step to destroy it.

There is so much I wish I had known before this whole adventure began. Before I'd even heard of weight-loss surgery, I was already a serial dieter, trying every idea, no matter how wacky.

I wasted my forties yo-yo dieting, and ended up with a worse problem than when I started out.

Heck, when I reached for my first diet, after baby number two or three, I was only about 10½ stone. I was a generous(!) size 12. The costume lady at Pebble Mill, where we made *Good Morning with Anne and Nick*, was mildly annoyed with me because I was stretching the buttons on my trousers. That was the start of it all. Yet 10 years later, and after a million wonder diets, I ended up at 15 stone 10. So much for diets!

OK, I know I must have been doing something wrong, like eating too much of the wrong stuff and sitting in front of a computer screen all day, but let's face it – the diets didn't help me. In fact, I think they made things worse.

I was really, really miserable about my weight. Depressed, even. Not about life – but very depressed about my weight. I got to the point where I thought nothing could be done. I was beginning to have the aches and pains that are generally suffered by the overweight. Niggling backaches, fat ankles at night, breathlessness...and I had high blood pressure. Was I going to develop diabetes? Would I keel over one day from a heart attack or stroke? Was I going to die younger than I should rightfully expect? Was I really increasing my risks of cancer?

You read the headlines, you hear the friendly GP on the morning news shows muttering something about increased risks, but you never really think she's talking about you, do you? Yet she certainly is.

I started to realise that this was not just about how I looked in the mirror, or even on TV. This was about my life. That's how important your body is. It is your life. You cannot be a mother, wife, career woman – or anything else at all in fact – if your body is compromised.

Me and my operation

At my lowest point I started Googling phrases such as 'stomach stapling' and 'jaw wiring' to see if there really might be an extreme, physical solution. Trouble was, all that came up were hair-raising stories about extraordinarily obese people. You know, the ones who can't move, and they have to knock a wall down to get them out on a forklift truck to take them to hospital. Surely, I thought, there must be something to help ordinary, run-of-the-mill fatties. People like me who were fairly normal in all other respects, and who weren't eating 10 pizzas a day and being bed-bathed by a small army of neighbours.

And that's when I heard from a friend of a friend of a friend who'd had a gastric band fitted – and the weight was apparently cascading off her. So I spoke to this friend of a friend of a friend and she was a sensible, sane, intelligent person. She was even a medical professional, so I thought – well, if she thinks it's OK, then it must be! She suggested I go to Belgium, where I could have the operation much more cheaply than in Britain, where the hospitals have no MRSA, and where they speak perfect English. I could do the whole trip on the Eurostar, so it would be quick, convenient and, I hoped, discreet.

I must confess, I didn't do any more research. I can barely believe it now, but I wanted to keep the whole thing entirely confidential. I thought, I'll have the op, I'll lose weight slowly and surely, and then my weight need never be an issue again.

So I rang the doctor direct, paid him his money, and hopped on the Eurostar at Waterloo one cold autumn morning. I met him for the first time that afternoon. He could speak English quite well, but frankly, his staff and nurses couldn't speak English at all. Now I'm not criticising them. I don't speak a word of Flemish! But when you're having an operation, it's nice to be able to chit-chat, ask questions, you know? Well, I never got the chance. It was just heads down and get on with it.

They weighed me, did some blood tests, measured me for elastic stockings and that was it. I went off back to the hotel for my last supper! I was really excited to think how everything would be different from that meal onward.

The next morning, however, I did feel a bit scared, so I took out my laptop and wrote letters to all my children. That was the wobbly time, when I thought: Has it really come to this? Am I such a dunce at dieting that I have come all this way, in secret, without even telling my family, to have elective surgery – to have a contraption put inside me to stop me eating too much?

Before I could have a total collapse of nerve, the theatre trolley arrived. Then I was out like a light.

After a painful and rather distressing experience in the recovery room, and an uncomfortable night with a weird pain in my shoulder (which I found out, six months later, was 'referred pain', common after laparoscopic surgery), I awoke the next morning feeling pretty good – and quite excited. A nutritionist popped in and gave me a couple of pages of dietary advice: I'd have to stick to fluids for two weeks, followed by two more weeks of puréed and mashed food, before returning to a normal diet. She kept saying that if I ate too much or too quickly, I might 'bring it over'. I looked quizzical. So she mimed it. She meant vomiting!

After that, the surgeon came in, said all had gone well, wished me luck and was gone. It hadn't exactly been a five-star experience, but it had been quick, efficient and straightforward, and I didn't think I'd been recognised by anyone. I stayed one more night in the nearby hotel, then came back home thinking everything would be different.

After the op

I stuck rigidly to the 'baby food' diet because I'd just had a major operation and, if truth be told, I was a little bit frightened. I was also becoming hideously aware that I was hundreds of miles away from my surgeon, should I cause myself problems, such as getting a piece of food stuck...

Four weeks later, though, and back on to solids, eating didn't feel different. I felt as hungry as before, and when I ate, I couldn't feel any restriction whatsoever. The days went by and still I hoped. But it was as though I had never had an operation. My weight stayed stubbornly the same. It was as though the band simply would not work.

I couldn't understand it. Only after weeks of Googling things did I find out that the band was adjustable and I should be going back to have what they call a 'fill'. This is where the surgeon injects some saline into the port to inflate the band and increase the restriction. My surgeon had not even mentioned it. I knew nothing about fills. So I rang him up.

'Ah yes, you might need a fill,' he agreed pleasantly.

Can I have one?

'But yes, of course,' he said helpfully.

Why didn't you mention this before? I asked. I've never even heard of a fill!

'Ah, well,' he soothed, 'some patients never need them...'

I am utterly horrified now that I went through the whole procedure without being told about fills. The aftercare to this operation is almost more important than the op itself, yet no mention had been made.

So I found myself back on the Eurostar – staying again at a local hotel because the surgeon wanted to see me early in the morning. Suddenly, the 'cheap option' of European surgery didn't seem quite so cheap. The costs were mounting steadily.

Next morning I experienced the mysterious fill. It's a surprisingly simple and quick process. The surgeon sticks a needle (quite painlessly) into the gastric band's port, just beneath your skin, and injects a little saline solution. You can feel the difference straight away. It feels a little like you're going to burp. Afterwards, I was asked to drink some water – just to make sure it wasn't too tight. When I managed that quite easily, he stopped and thought. 'Maybe I should put a little more in?' he asked.

So in went the needle again, and he squeezed a little more saline into the port just underneath my skin. I drank again, and this time I could feel a restriction as the water went down. It took five minutes to drink a cup of water. At first he was anxious that the band was too tight, but eventually he relaxed.

'I would not want to fill any more – this is very tight indeed.' Then he beamed enthusiastically. 'You will lose a lot of weight, I think!' I smiled too. At last this thing was going to work.

'Fifty euros, please' he said. 'Very cheap! I'll take any currency.'

That's health tourism. An operation is a commodity – no different than an iPod or a digital camera. You get what you pay for and no more. Who am I to complain? I thought. I've got what I wanted – a gastric band. Now with this fill, it will start to work and I will lose weight.

But once I was home and eating normally, nothing happened. No sense of restriction, no weight loss – nothing. I felt awful.

I went back again – for another fill. This time, he said, it was really tight – he wouldn't be able to get much more saline in. I thought, I must have a very thin stomach.

Yet back home there was still little change in the way I could eat. Bandsters, as they call gastric band patients, shouldn't really be able to eat a piece of bread or, say, a banana without feeling that it's too much. I'd heard other patients boast that one glass of orange juice made them feel full. But still I felt no fullness, zero satisfaction, and only the tiniest hint of restriction. And please believe me, I really was not melting down Mars bars. I was eating healthily – pitta breads, tuna salads, fruit and veggies.

I've done this before, I thought. I'm a sucker for gadgets – got a house full of them. This time, though, I've been really stupid. I've bought into a gadget that's actually been placed inside me – and it doesn't work.

I'd gone all the way to Belgium, had all the worry, all the fear, all the expense of this operation and had nothing to show for it save a few little scars on my belly and a large hole in the bank balance. Was it the band that was useless or me? Was I the only person in the world for whom even surgery didn't work? I just concluded, as all fatties do, that *I* was a failure – it was all my fault. I was going to be a 60-year-old fat lady after all, which is what I really dreaded.

And that's when *Celebrity Fit Club* came along.

Celebrity Fit Club

Oh, horror of horrors. Now this is getting difficult to write again… my stomach's feeling queasy. Perhaps I should go and make myself a cup of coffee? Or spring-clean the house? Or start a marathon bake and fill the freezer with home-made bread and muffins? Because this is a really painful bit. *Celebrity Fit Club*. Even the mention of it makes me break out in a cold sweat.

What a horror of a programme. What a bunch of bastards (well, some of them). What a giant waste of air time. What exploitation cynically disguised as 'health programming'. There are names I will never forget from those days. They're on a little list that I'll be giving to St Peter at the Pearly Gates (when I ever get there, hope-fully not for a very long time!) – and I'll be saying, 'You might want to refuse this mealy-mouthed bunch...'

Oh, that's better. I'm angry again now. I can write.

You might ask – and quite reasonably – why on earth did I agree to take part? Because it held out the last glimmer of hope for me. The producers promised me it was all about fun, together-ness and teamwork, and would give me unprecedented access to the top weight-loss experts in the world. Every contestant who'd ever been on before had lost stones in weight, they promised. It always works!

On the other hand, I wondered, can I really stand on scales on public TV every Saturday night? Well, I thought, maybe that sort of public humiliation would be the kick up the butt I needed. So I agreed to do it. I didn't tell them I had a gastric band inside me because by then it was irrelevant.

Now if *Big Brother* taught me that fat is the one last permissible prejudice, then *Fit Club* taught me another quite shocking lesson: that the majority of weight-loss experts are bullies, particularly in the media, and believe that there is only one way to lose weight and get fit – and that's by suffering. So when I confessed to having a gastric band inside me, which was, by the way, demonstrably *not* working, they pounced on me with all the bigotry of a McCarthy witch-hunt.

Silly, ignorant people were allowed to turn the whole matter into headline-grabbing opportunism. Something about accusing me of cheating. Duh? I wasn't even losing weight. But never mind the facts – just try anything to better the ratings (which were al-ready poor, and continued to fall). Let's rip Anne to pieces; that should make a front page or two. And then we'll beg her to stay in the show just so we can do it all again next week. We'll even get

Dale Winton (the show's host) to ring her and beg her to come back. That should do the trick.

I was polite to Dale when he rang. I shouldn't have been. I should have told him where to stuff his mobile phone.

Just the memory of *Fit Club* still makes my skin crawl. But it taught me a lot about attitudes.

Putting things right

If I'd been low before my surgery, I was at rock bottom after escaping from *Fit Club*. I couldn't have coped without the support of family and friends. But then I got a call from an unexpected quarter: a private medical company here in Britain that specialises in cosmetic surgery and obesity surgery. They said they couldn't understand why my band wasn't working. Would I like to find out why? We agreed to meet.

First things first, they advised – we need to have a look at your band. So I was whisked off for an X-ray. And that X-ray proved I hadn't got what I bargained for. My gastric band was in the wrong place. There it was, large as life on the big screen. The surgeon, Shaw Somers, pointed it all out to me. (Shaw is one of Britain's most experienced bariatric, or obesity, surgeons. He's done literally hundreds of bands and bypasses. You might have seen him on Discovery Health's *Fat Doctor*.)

My band had not been positioned around the top part of the stomach, as gastric bands should be. It had been placed, like a loose collar, around the base of the oesophagus, where it meets the top of the stomach. It wasn't around the stomach at all. And it wasn't even stitched in place, as it should be!

'That's not where it's designed to go,' said Shaw, shaking his head. 'But I have seen this before, I'm afraid. I am honestly getting a bit fed up with having to repair botched operations done in Europe on the cheap.'

I couldn't believe it. There it was, this wretched band, sitting in the wrong place. And I'd been through all this bloody misery – feeling a rotten failure, going through the hell of *Celebrity Fit Club* – because the darned Belgian surgeon had put the thing in the wrong place. Why did he do that?

Well, apparently it's a much quicker and easier operation that allows them to do more ops per day. It seems that some people do lose weight with it because the band may give them a feeling of restriction when they swallow. But the oesophagus isn't meant to take that sort of strain, and it must be painful. So they might be losing weight because it's painful to eat, and they might even develop a fear of food. That's not what the band is designed to do. I've even checked that with the band manufacturers.

Once I'd got over the shock and then past the anger, I had to make a decision. Should I have the thing taken out or have the band repositioned? It was terribly distressing. I'd been upset enough just going through elective surgery once. I had tortured myself with thoughts of the risks – what if I died on the operating table and left my kids motherless? How would they feel to have lost a mother just because she couldn't lose weight the traditional way?

Since my operation, there have been several cases in the news telling that very story. They are horrendously tragic, yet I do believe they demonstrate the heartbreaking dilemma being faced by more and more men and women.

Should I try again, take the risk of another surgery, or resign myself to obesity and all the likely health risks?

I suppose there was one other choice – to keep trying to lose weight through exercise and diets. I could go on punishing myself and feeling depressed every time I failed for another 10 years.

Ultimately, I still wanted what I had bought into, so I had the operation all over again – this time in London. I had a surgeon I could talk to, nurses who were friendly, family and friends around me, and it was an enjoyable and positive experience. This time, when I ate I felt full quickly and I physically couldn't consume any more. I would sit in a restaurant and happily watch the waiter take away my plate after I'd eaten just a quarter of my meal, knowing I couldn't force down another morsel even if I'd wanted to.

The weight dropped off and I was thrilled. I reduced by a dress size a month and lost about 3 stone before my weight reached a plateau, and now I'm having to work hard to keep the momentum going. It's frustrating, but it's better than being 15 stone 10 lb.

Since my surgery

One of the biggest side effects of having gastric band surgery is an enormous swelling of...the mailbag. Well, it certainly was in my case! And I am sure it has been the same for Fern Britton, or Sharon Osbourne, or countless others with famous names, who have, like it or not, become linked with obesity surgery.

Even nearly two years on, I am still set upon by large ladies (and a few blokes) in Marks & Spencer and John Lewis, who approach me, beaming: 'Are you Anne Diamond? Haven't you done well!', and then grasp my elbow and drag me behind a clothes rail to whisper more pressing questions:

'Where did you get it done?'

'How do I know I'll get a good surgeon?'

'What is it like to eat?'

'Aren't you sick all the time?'

'How fat do you have to be?'

'What can I do? My doctor won't even talk to me about it...'

That's when I realised I had to spread the word; not because obesity surgery is for everyone – it most certainly is not – but because desperate people need to know the real facts. And you cannot get across the true facts, warts and all, in a quickie TV interview, or even in a newspaper or magazine feature – where they invariably get something wrong. I don't know how many times I have read that I had my stomach 'stapled', when in fact the band operation was the stapling alternative. There are also such shocking headlines about the risks, which often don't fully explain what happened and why. Nor do they show any understanding of the complex emotional and physical circumstances that lead someone to put themselves 'under the knife' rather than stay obese.

I myself was appalled to read 'Anne Diamond Stomach Op Killed My Girl' in the *Daily Mirror* one morning, about a 25-year-old woman who'd had a gastric band fitted, successfully lost a great deal of weight, and then died a couple of years later. The headline blamed the operation before the inquest had even been held.

Of course there are risks, and people should know them, but always in the context of their circumstances. Obesity is, after all, one of the top risk factors for surgery anyway, so when you talk about bariatric surgery, you are already talking about an extraordinarily high-risk group. But individuals have to weigh that against their own precarious health prognosis.

What's more, I knew people needed to know the facts so that they could make an informed decision – and perhaps even reject the whole idea. But where was the forum for such a discussion?

My roadshow

I decided to grasp the nettle, and in the spring of 2007, still very much a slimming 'work in progress' myself, I took my show on the road, speaking at Manchester, Birmingham and Leeds, along with a panel of surgeons, health experts, surgery providers and Louise Diss, a representative from TOAST (The Obesity Aware-nesss and Solutions Trust), who'd once been obese herself and had lost about 10 stone without resorting to surgery.

I met some truly wonderful people in those audiences. And I learnt a lot too about the unique set of men and women I was addressing. For a start, don't hold a gathering about obesity surgery upstairs...

My Manchester gig was on the first floor of Manchester Town Hall, right at the top of a huge flight of magnificent stone stairs. One lady met me afterwards and told me she'd missed much of my talk because it had taken her nearly all evening just to get up the steps. She walked breathlessly, with two sticks, and tears were streaming down her face both with the effort and the emotion that had driven her so far.

'I'm dying and I know it,' she gasped. 'I just can't seem to do anything about my weight. I have tried absolutely everything, for years. I have come here because I think surgery is going to be my only lifeline – but Anne,' and she grasped my hand tight, 'I just can't afford it. I have asked my doctor and he says I need surgery but the NHS won't pay for it where I live. Is there anything I can do?' Then she sat down and started to cry. I thought, where are they now, those callous people who like to spit: 'It's not rocket sci-ence, you know. All you have to do is eat less and exercise more.'

This is a subject we'd already covered that night with the ex-pert panel. I was able to lead her over to one of the northwest's top bariatric surgeons, who sat down with her and started to write out names and addresses for her, and coached her on what to say, how to say it, and to whom. That's when you get that feeling – that if you have helped just one person get their life back, then it's all been worthwhile. But there were loads more.

One couple, very well-to-do and informed, had been sitting right at the front of my Leeds night, shaking their heads, nodding, and asking some very articulate questions. I remember thinking: I wonder why they're here? Neither of them looked particularly overweight. In fact, they were researching for their adult son. They were worried about him.

'He's rich, successful and he's got everything he could ever want, but his health,' they confided in me afterwards. 'He is very, very overweight. We don't want him to die like that; we want him to live!'

Another stick-thin lady was at the Birmingham session with her very, very large daughter – a beautiful girl whose childhood, you could see, was escaping her. They'd tried everything and just ended up more upset, more depressed and more frightened for the future.

In the corner two big guys, who spent all night summoning up the courage to speak, revealed heartbreaking stories about how their weight was affecting their lives.

I don't think anyone was there on a whim, or because they were seeking an easy way out of their plight. Many confessed that even the full and frank discussion had done little to ease their fear of surgery, and they knew they'd never be able to do it.

At the first Manchester gig, where my expert surgeon was the eminent Professor Mike McMahon, I was surprised when I thought I heard heckling. It was actually a very bubbly, slim blonde at the back, who simply couldn't contain herself. She stood up and called out: 'I want to say thank you to the prof! He's given me back my body and my life. I had a band two years ago and I've lost 8 stone – and I would never have done it without him!'

I called the series of evenings my 'Get Your Life Back' tour. I wish we'd been able to do more. Not because I want everyone to have surgery – I don't. It's just not suitable for many, and others simply can't face the surgeon's knife. It doesn't even work for everyone – but if you have been fighting a losing battle with obesity and your health is at risk, you need to know the facts – from the experts, and perhaps from someone like me, who has been through it herself.

This was the gist of my message:

* Obesity surgery is serious stuff – and you need to know *all* the facts.
* No one goes into it lightly.
* It's not cosmetic surgery – and it really is not about wanting to come out of the hospital looking like Jordan.

I have now met hundreds of surgery patients who have had varying amounts of success with their gastric bands and gastric bypasses, and none of them went under the knife on an impulse. It is about finding a way to stop you being obese or dangerously overweight. It is about being fit and healthy. It is about getting your life back, rediscovering the real you inside.

No matter what the adverts suggest, a gastric band or a bypass cannot turn you into Catherine Zeta Jones and propel you to Hollywood and a nice rich husband. But it can help you lose the weight that's tying you down, compromising your health and your future. The rest you have to do yourself.

Real life

In the USA there's a big TV star called Star Jones. She certainly is a star. She's an African-American lawyer who became a co-anchor on *The View*, one of the most watched TV programmes in America, where a panel of women air their opinions about anything and everything. (It's like *The Wright Stuff*, but all girls!)

And she was big – once. She became especially controversial when she started losing weight – quite dramatically losing over 10 stone almost in front of everyone's eyes. At first she denied she'd had surgery, then later she confirmed that she'd had a gastric bypass. (Sound familiar?) She said she'd denied it at first because she didn't want to become a poster girl for a medical procedure that could have tragic consequences for someone else.

Later, on *Larry King Live*, CNN's famous chat show, she showed off her new slim figure. And she looked utterly fabulous – slim, toned, curvy in all the right places, and downright sexy.

But she stressed that the gastric band doesn't give you the body – it just helps you to lose weight and get more healthy. 'You want this kinda body, you have to work damn hard for it!'

And what Star says needs stressing over and over again – to the media and to those who think weight-loss surgery is about vanity, and is a 'quick fix' or an easy option.

❝ Surgery provides a weight-loss tool – nothing more. ❞

The lowdown on gastric band ops

Nothing quite prepares you for your first time as an observer inside an operating theatre, especially if you're witnessing a surgical procedure that you have actually undergone. You gaze at the body on the table and you see yourself. You watch the surgeon slice through the skin and fat, and you imagine your own blood dripping from the wound. You gawp as he punctures the patient's belly with what seem like brutal pieces of laparoscopic equipment. And you wince and wonder at the surgeon's skill and strength, and the resilience of the human body.

I'm not squeamish about blood and guts, thank goodness. In a gastric banding operation there isn't much blood at all, and all the guts stay inside anyway because nearly all such operations are done through a 'keyhole'. So I was thrilled when one of the UK's leading bariatric surgeons invited me to witness the procedure everyone's talking about. Roger Ackroyd works in the Leeds area and is a veteran of about 2000 such operations, which makes him uniquely experienced.

'More bariatric surgeons are coming on line, but it will take time before they are up and running,' he told me as we scrubbed in. 'Until we train more, there are only about 10 truly experienced surgeons in the UK, and we are all working flat out!'

I met his patient beforehand – a lovely mid-30s mum of two, whom I will call Katie, who was pinning all her hopes on a gastric band to wage her personal war on fat. She'd finally had enough of serial dieting when she regained the 6 stone she had lost on a long and intensive meal replacement programme. She'd heard my story in the media and vowed she'd learn from my mistakes. Even though it was expensive (some £8000), she decided to have the op near her home town, with a surgeon she could easily contact, and whose reputation was, she said quite simply, 'the best'!

She would have been impressed by his dexterity, though perhaps also daunted by how quickly we all become just a slab of meat once the anaesthetic has knocked us out. Did I look like that on the operating table? I wondered. Just a big blob with weird instruments sticking out of five incisions in my belly? The theatre staff had, of course, seen it all before many times, and just got on with their jobs. I crept closer to take it all in. Into one incision, Roger inserted a plastic nozzle through which carbon dioxide was blown into the stomach, inflating it like a flesh balloon. This was to give him room inside to manoeuvre his instruments. Another tiny incision was for a camera and another for a clamp to hold the liver out of the way. Two were for the instruments in each hand, and the largest one, where the carbon dioxide had entered, was where the gastric band's port would be placed. This is the access point, sewn just beneath the skin, where the surgeon can later inject saline in order to tighten the band. (The tighter the band, the harder it is for food to pass into the stomach, so the less you eat.)

I'd always imagined such an operation taking at least 35–40 minutes. In fact, it took Roger less than 20. He twiddled away with his implements, rather like a woman knitting a baby's bootee with overlong size 20 needles through a letterbox. In went the silicone band through one hole. Something very like a long crochet needle picked it up inside and wound it around the stomach. You could watch everything on a monitor as Roger deftly stitched the band in place. Then it was all over, Katie was whisked away into the recovery room, and within minutes she was a human being again, regaining consciousness and being reassured all had gone well.

'It's not the perfect answer to the obesity problem, but it is an effective one,' Roger told me later. 'Of course, I look forward to the day when we can, as a society, get our act together and stop the spread of obesity. It would put me out of work, but I'd welcome it. I don't think it's going to happen soon, though.'

Other types of surgery

In the UK, as elsewhere in the world, the gastric band and gastric bypass are the most common types of surgery recommended to treat obesity, but only as a last resort. Another procedure is the gastric balloon, which is passed down into the stomach via the throat and inflated inside to make the patient feel full and thus eat less. This is generally used for six months at the most, and then has to be removed. Medical companies claim it teaches you how to change your eating behaviours, but many surgeons are sceptical, and patients often complain that they regain weight as soon as it is removed. That's true of the gastric band, which is intended to stay in for life. In studies where patients have had bands removed, they have nearly always regained their lost weight.

There are other procedures too, including the sleeve gastrectomy and the duodenal switch, neither of which is commonly practised in the UK.

In 2006, NICE, the National Institute for Health and Clinical Excellence, which advises whether treatments should be provided by the NHS, recommended surgery for anyone with a BMI (see page 77) of over 40. They also advised that surgery should be available for anyone with a BMI of over 35 if their obesity was causing 'significant disease', such as type 2 diabetes or high blood pressure, and if they had tried everything else on offer and had still failed to lose weight. That doesn't automatically mean you can get surgery on the NHS, though. It's a 'postcode lottery', depending on where you live. Even in those areas where it is possible to have the operation free, many Primary Care Trusts (PCTs) restrict surgery to those with a much higher BMI, such as 45 or 50.

A gastric band operation usually requires just one night in hospital. A bypass is a much, much bigger deal: the patient goes into the High Dependency Unit, with drips, drains and a tube up the nose, and spends about four further days in bed. Although there are a number of variations in the latter surgery, the most commonly done are the roux-en-y gastric bypass (RGB) and biliopancreatic diversion (BPD). Both change the normal process of digestion by making the stomach smaller and allowing food to bypass part of the small intestine so that you absorb fewer calories and nutrients. That's why bypass patients have to take extra vitamins for the rest of their life. They can never eat anything sweet again either, or they experience what's called 'dumping syndrome', whereby the body protests at both ends, and they have to lie down for a couple of hours.

Bariatric surgery is only for those who've exhausted everything else. No matter how hard the sell — and some commercial companies and medical providers do give the impression that obesity surgery is as 'easy' and 'desirable' as cosmetic surgery — it is risky, requiring a general anaesthetic to a patient already deemed 'high risk' because of their obesity. I personally worry that the band is being 'oversold'. There are about four different types of band available at the moment, and they are fiercely marketed. What they don't flag up is that between 2 and 5 per cent of band patients end up being dissatisfied and go back after a couple of years, asking for a 'revision' to a bypass. It's an expensive reality check because a band (at the time of writing) will cost you about £8000, and a conversion to a bypass (which involves removing the band first) can cost an *additional* £11,000–£12,000. In the UK a bypass operation will generally cost about £10,000. It pays to talk things through with your surgeon, and together choose the right operation for you. Changing your mind later could be very costly.

CHAPTER 1

FAT IS A
FOUR-LETTER WORD

*

Oh, yes – fat really is a four-letter word because nowadays it's almost the biggest insult you can hurl at anyone. And it hurts.

Calling someone 'fat' is not just a plain statement of fact – it's a moral judgement. You're saying, 'You are someone who is morally bankrupt; you're useless, pathetic, out of control and a failure.' In our modern culture, for a celebrity to be fat, well – that's one of the biggest sins on the planet. Loudmouths in the press, and even many ordinary people who are probably quite kindly in other respects, see it as inexcusable and treat it with utter contempt. You get the feeling they'd be nicer to murderers and paedophiles.

'Fired for Being FAT! Kirstie's Diet Meltdown!' screamed one headline about *Cheers* star Kirstie Alley.

'Oprah's 48-hour Food Binge!'

'And the Weight Goes On! Lonely Cher Piles on 26 Pounds!'

'Big Fat Liar!' about Fern Britton when her gastric band came to light. She hadn't actually lied, by the way.

'Skeletal Spice!' about Victoria Beckham. Ooops! Okay, so it's not about fat – but the lack of it is still fodder for the tabloids, and the vitriol is just as scathing. It just shows that the media has body dysmorphia, never mind the people it discusses day in, day out.

Maybe it's funny for the headline writers, who are all, presumably, picture perfect. When you are the subject of their bile, it's not funny at all – you never get used to it, and yes, it really does hurt. And what sort of effect does it have on us as a society?

Should we be surprised that a whole generation of teenagers is suffering from eating disorders, ranging from out-of-control obesity to an obsession with dieting pills and anorexia?

Celebrity Big Brother

When I came out of the *Celebrity Big Brother* house, back in 2002, it was the first time the British public, and particularly the press, had seen the Bigger Me. I had been known as the Elfin Queen of Breakfast Television, and subsequently as the pert Queen of Daytime, who still managed to keep a trim figure despite being a mum five times over... I spent the four years after that in radio (where I presented the LBC breakfast show with Sir Nick Lloyd and later with Tommy Boyd – eating hot buttered toast in between interviews) and bringing up my children at our home in Oxfordshire. No one, least of all me, realised I had put on a fair bit of weight until I turned up at Elstree Studios with my *Big Brother* silver suitcase and chirruped some ridiculously hearty answers to Davina McCall's showbizzy questions. I think of it now like that scene from the Woody Allen movie *Annie Hall*, where the conversation is one long, embarrassing platitude – and the real meanings are hovering underneath in subtitles:

Davina: How do you think you're going to cope being locked up in a house with five other celebrities?

Me: It's going to be fun. I like meeting people and I'm a professional interviewer, so it shouldn't be hard getting to know them!

Subtitle: I'm already hating it, so just let me get in there and get it over with...

Davina: Why do you want to take part in this second series of *Celebrity Big Brother*?

Me: Because it's for charity and one should never turn down an adventure!

Subtitle: Because my agent told me I must – to remind people that I'm still alive!

Davina: How long do you think you're going to last in there?

Me: As long as it takes. I'll just have lots of fun and see what happens.

Subtitle: Please let me be first out or I just might kill myself...

I am so glad I didn't see my own image as I waddled down the runway, wheeling my suitcase behind me, and up the chrome stairs into the house. I had deliberately chosen a trouser suit with a long cardigan to hide my posterior. But nothing really hides a big bum because anything baggy just turns you into an ambling tent. So that was me – a big, blue, knitted wigwam with a steely grin on top.

I didn't see that video, or the other horrible images of me, until I was let out some six days later. (In those days, that was a long time inside the *Big Brother* house. It certainly felt like hard labour.)

Had I read the fattist, sizeist coverage of my appearance, I might have thrown myself off the roof.

'Sad, Lonely and Desperate' was one *Daily Mail* headline, based on absolutely nothing but my size.

'Anne Diamond's kids must be ashamed to have a mother with such a gargantuan backside,' wrote Lynda Lee-Potter.

And every picture they printed was of me eating. I had no more to eat than anyone else in the house – in fact, food was a scarce commodity because we had to earn it by completing special tasks at which we were pretty useless. But hey, that's so-called reality television. It gets heavily edited, and then the picture editors choose the best way to illustrate their story. That's the name of the game. Can't really complain? Except about the astonishing truth that fat is clearly the last permissible prejudice in this new, politically correct world.

IN DEFENCE OF FERN

Only ignorant, unfeeling snobs would call TV presenter Fern Britton a cheat for getting a gastric band to sort out her body. Just a short time ago we all loved her for her new, healthy look and her radiant face. So what's changed since her dramatic revelation? She still looks wonderful, is now much healthier and less likely to suffer from diabetes, heart disease, stroke or even cancer, and her life has probably been extended by some 10 years. If I were a member of her family, I would give her a big hug for the brave step she took – to finally do something about the life-threatening condition she was suffering from. Just think of her kids. I know what they'd say – same as mine: 'We love you, Mum, and anything that makes you healthier and happier is OK by us!'

Obesity is a killer, let's have no doubt about that. It's not a sign of being lazy or stupid – it's a sign of the times. Any woman in TV knows that more than most. The camera over-emphasises every extra pound of flesh, while the pressure to look skinny is almost unbearable. We live in a world where the worst sort of food is peddled to us like drugs, yet we are lambasted if we dare put on a pound or two. We live busy, stressful lives, and some of us are predisposed to put on weight more than others. That's a fact.

What's more, we have allowed the media to dictate how obesity should be tackled – and up has sprung a questionable diet industry and a clutch of so-called weight-loss experts who have become rich by bullying us into submission. They say there's only one way to lose weight, and that's through suffering and deprivation. You've got to feel the pain because you have 'let yourself go'. That's the whole attitude of the media – and it's absolute rubbish. I say, 'Well done, Fern, for finding another way.'

Instead, some people choose to wag their disapproving finger at her and call her a liar. But she hasn't lied. She might have been selective about how much information she chose to make public, but who can blame her? After the abuse that was hurled at me when I disclosed that I had had a gastric band operation, I for one fully understand.

It's a fallacy to say she didn't achieve her new look through exercise and healthy eating – that is exactly what the gastric band helps you to achieve. It's a tool, nothing else. It is neither a magic pill nor the 'easy option' some of the adverts would have you believe. It's like having a corset – on your insides! Like the ultimate portion controller, it simply restricts the volume of what you can eat, but it does not stop you secretly bingeing on chocolate, meringues, mousses, ice cream, hoummous or mayonnaise. They all slip through the band like syrup, as do fattening alcohol and mixers, so any idea that you don't have to use will-power and determination is a gross misunderstanding of what the gastric band is all about.

But it is not for everyone, and with some patients, it will never work. Neither will it sort out your head. Since I had it, I have discovered new facts about what is a treatment in its infancy. The gastric band suits only 'volume eaters'. If you're the sort who's addicted to sweets and chocolates, you'll sabotage yourself from the beginning. And if you live in a fat family, with a bulging biscuit tin and a fridge full of junk, you'll end up fat and frustrated.

The idea is that the band helps you to make the right decisions and, hopefully, develop healthier habits. Nothing Fern has done with her band negates anything she has said, or even done with her Ryvita adverts and her Pilates video. Leave her alone to enjoy her well-deserved slimness. But be warned if you think it's for you – do your research first. Despite the headlines, it is not a fast-track ticket to losing weight.

Fat is a workplace issue

You can call someone a big fat pig and no one will stop you – not even the law. Unbelievably, in the UK you can be refused a job because of your size. There's no law preventing discrimination on the grounds of obesity.

❝ In a recent survey 30 per cent of human resources bosses said that they believed obesity was a valid medical reason for not employing some-one. What's more, a whopping 93 per cent of them said they would hire a 'normal weight' applicant as opposed to an obese one if they were otherwise identically qualified. ❞

This was highlighted for many people, and particularly me, when the following case came to light.

Real life

Marie Parker, at 4 feet 11 inches and 12 stone, has been driving school buses in Gloucestershire for 20 years, and even won commendations from the Department of Transport. Then she wanted to move to Northern Ireland, so she applied for a job with a different bus company, TransLink. On the form they asked for her weight and height. They calculated her BMI as 34.1, so refused even to interview her. They said their drivers had to be medically fit and healthy, and, based on her BMI, Marie wasn't.

I met Marie on a radio programme. She put her case quite bluntly. She wasn't fat. She was a good bus driver – in fact, she'd actually won some awards. She was hurt and upset that she hadn't even been given an interview.

I was shocked for her too. When I looked at her picture on the BBC website I could quite clearly see that she wasn't really fat. It's just not how most ordinary people would describe her. I was dumbfounded when I realised that her BMI was about the same as mine. I've never driven a bus, but I would hate to think that someone could classify me as too fat to do so. And if, at that point, I was too fat to drive a bus for TransLink, how come I could safely drive my children around in our 'people carrier'?

Duncan Bannatyne, a famous entrepreneur and one of the 'dragons' on TV's *Dragon's Den*, has said: 'Fat people don't work as hard as people who are not fat.' He expanded in an interview: 'I think somebody who's fit can think faster and work faster. Somebody who hasn't looked after themselves won't train their brain, won't train their body, will just smoke cigarettes or stuff themselves with pies. They're less likely to go out and want to apply themselves and work hard.'

You see how the stereotype is reinforced? I wonder whether Duncan Bannatyne has ever seen anyone fat 'stuff themselves with pies', yet the image is clearly quite vivid in his mind. 'Pies' equals Homer Simpson, laziness and greed. Interestingly, replace the word 'pie' with 'sandwich' or 'biscuit' and immediately the harshness of the statement softens.

Everyone assumes, if you're fat, that you gorge on chips and cheeseburgers. When I made a serious film report about gastric bands for the BBC, and while my voice-over was detailing obesity statistics, they underlaid pictures of French fries and fast food.

The assumption is always made by slim people – who may well eat as much, if not more, rubbish food – and this automatic supposition is an insult. In fact, as discusssed later on, all the obesity doctors I interviewed around the world said that it doesn't take much to make you fat:

❝ *Just a daily biscuit added to your usual intake over a year can tip the scales from 'normal' to 'overweight', or 'overweight' to 'obese'. Just one daily cookie.* **❞**

While the dragon might have dared to breathe such fire, even at the risk of burning his own clients, hundreds of big bosses feel the same way. According to the journal *Personnel Today*, which last year asked me to write a response to its survey because it was so shocking, 79 per cent of UK bosses believe there is prejudice against people who are seriously overweight, and 70 per cent think overweight people are regarded as lacking self-discipline. So they're aware there is a problem for a huge proportion of their employees, even if they think it's self-inflicted.

Elspeth Watt, director of the training and development organisation Calibre HR & Training, put it another way: 'Obese people are often thought of as lazy or incapable of working to the same level, whereas in reality, weight frequently has nothing to do with performance. This will become an increasingly key issue for employers. Equally, I hope, attitudes will start to change.'

So should fat people in the workplace be ignored, shunned or supported? And when does support become patronising, nannying or even bullying? Does mere acknowledgment of the obese among us amount to discrimination? How would we feel if a personnel or human resources officer took us aside at work one day and told us:

1   You are overweight.
2   You are now enrolled on the company's 'Get Fit and Healthy' programme.

I know I'd probably blow a fuse and then go home and cry. Rather like when a girlfriend bought me a pair of naughty knickers for my fiftieth birthday – they were lovely but...they were a size 18. She was only being realistic, but I was mortified.

So what's a responsible employer to do? Seventy-five per cent of them don't know – they just feel they should be doing something.

Enter a whole new industry of people advising big corporations, and even councils, how to encourage a healthier lifestyle in their workforce – and the deals are worth millions. New companies, such as Nuffield Proactive Health, have sprung up to put fitness and health at the top of the agenda for big city businesses. Underlying their whole enterprise is a belief that fat is bad for productivity.

'The number of overweight people has increased by 400 per cent in the past 25 years,' says Nuffield Health's chief executive Chris Jessop. 'People are leading increasingly sedentary lifestyles, and employees who are seriously overweight are less productive and have more sickness absence. It's a harsh fact, but it's true.'

The fat controllers

It's not only the workplace that harbours harsh attitudes to fat. The one place you might expect to go and get succour rather than scorn is the doctor's surgery. Yet the medical establishment, particularly the first line of primary care, the GP's surgery, can be the biggest barrier to practical help.

'I went to my doctor for help when I'd tried every diet in Britain, and he told me that I must be lazy and greedy – in so many words,' Chrissie told me. She's a midwife and one of my online buddies. She knows all the theory – she just can't put it into practice for herself.

'He stood in front of me on the scales and jiggled his own belly,' she complained. 'He was more obese than me, yet he seemed happy to pontificate about my weight. He told me there was only one way to lose weight – to eat less and exercise more. And then he laughed when I asked about diet pills and Xenical. He refused me any.

'"Believe me, if there was an easy way, don't you think I would do it?" he laughed at me. And so I left, with nothing, and feeling completely helpless and even more of a failure.'

Doctors aren't perfect. That's something you learn with age, I think. Some of them are fantastically clever and others are enlightened and inspired. But a few are a menace. I've been around long enough to meet all sorts.

The cot death campaign, which I led in the 1990s following the death of my son, Sebastian, taught me that doctors are good and bad – same as in any profession. In the decades preceding the 'Back to Sleep' campaign, it's clear that some doctors were complacent, condescending, arrogant and even ignorant about cot death. They accepted its occurrence as an intrinsic sadness that accompanied the routine business of childbirth. One learned professor (and I know others who supported his view) made up his own mind that multiple cot deaths *must* be murder (Frith 2003). Some seized control over post-mortem tissue and never even thought of telling parents that they were withholding their children's brains, lungs, livers and hearts for future examination. History has taught us that these views and actions were reprehensible.

Now, in the 21st century, the medical profession has to rid itself of an intrinsic hatred of fatties. In several studies reported in the American medical journal *Obesity Research*, doctors in the USA and UK were asked to give (anonymously) their attitude towards fat patients. More than half used derogatory terms, such as 'weak-willed, ugly, awkward, non-compliant, lazy, lacking in self-control, unsuccessful, unintelligent, dishonest', and then moaned about how they were 'put off' examining them, or couldn't fit a blood pressure cuff around their arms. Surgeons complained about having to cut through inches of 'blubber', and one clinician wrote: 'We have patients that make Jabba the Hutt look svelte.' Several members of BuddyPower have recounted appalling tales of cruelty from their own GPs and weight-loss clinics:

Real lives

'My GP is obese herself! She just gave me a lecture on how you can be fat and fit – and all I should do is eat organic. Complaining to her about my lifelong battle with weight felt like I was insulting her, and it all got horribly embarrassing. I just left thinking – well, if she knows all the health facts, and she is an intelligent, high-achieving woman, and she is fat herself, how am *I* ever going to beat it? I asked her about surgery and she laughed. I asked her about diet pills and she scoffed. It's like she was saying: "You're fat, learn to live with it!" But I can't. I hate myself. If I'd gone into her surgery moaning about depression, she would have given me pills for that. Yet ask for help with weight loss, and there is no help – just a blank wall.'

'I came out of my doctor's surgery crying. He more or less told me I was lying when I said that I really had tried to lose weight. Honestly, I can eat a couple of lettuce leaves and I put on weight. But he said I had to be "cheating" and he kept trying to taunt me into a confession. It was like I was on trial. I'll never go back to him again, but what am I going to do? I need help but no one's interested. No wonder people just go on the Internet and go off to Belgium or whatever to get a gastric band or a bypass – at least they don't have to go through unhelpful GPs like mine! It's my 40th birthday soon and I am dreading it. I am going to be fat and 40, and I need a party dress, but no matter how much I spend, it will still look like a tent. Why are tears so easy to shed, but weight so hard?'

One woman living in Seattle, USA, said doctors' attitudes were the main reason she started a fat acceptance group called SeaFattle. From early childhood she'd tried every diet under the sun. Most of these diets advised checking with her doctor first, so she always did.

'The craziest one was a diet that a friend of mine found when we were both 19. It was called Dr Linn's Diet, aka the Last Chance Diet. It was the forerunner to the Cambridge, Optifast and other liquid diets that are still around. But on this one you consumed 100 per cent protein – no fats, no carbohydrates at all – in the form of a thick, nasty-tasting liquid made from processed cowhides, sold under the uninviting name of Predigested Liquid Protein. I did this with my family doctor's approval and his minimal supervision. When I asked him what he thought of it he said: "Well, it's starvation, but a little starvation won't hurt you – it's better than being fat."

'With a doctor like that, who needs enemies?'

Another buddy from my website has an equally dim view of GPs and their grip on the obesity epidemic:

'...the government and press spend all this time and effort (and money) publicising how we have an obesity issue and how to help it. We have healthfood shows thrown under our noses and basically the "obesity epidemic" is a nationwide problem according to pretty much every newspaper and magazine you read.

'Yet my GPs (there have been many) clearly do not read or receive any of this literature. The best I have ever been offered by my GPs is pills. They have always readily handed out any slimming pill I asked for, from Xenical to Reductil.

'I recently went to my GP for advice after my failed gastric balloon and was put back on Reductil. This did not work. I have now changed my GP and arranged a gastric band in Belgium. My doctor was negative about this. (I know you have had a bad experience in Belgium.) She said I was not heavy enough for a gastric band at 18 stone 4. She was entirely unhelpful, and yet again tried to get me to take pills.

'When asked about counselling, she told me that I had managed to make the arrangements for my gastric band myself and pay for it, and suggested I go on the Internet and get some private counselling.

'Clearly the entire UK is aware of the so-called obesity epidemic, but not general practitioners. Am I the only person who feels like this or do I just have a bad experience with my doctors?

'I might add that one of my concerns when I went to my doctor was that I have (much to my shame) taken recreational drugs. I asked my doctor how this would affect me regarding anaesthetic, and she told me to speak to the anaesthetist. Again, I am not proud of what I have done, but as someone who clearly has addictive problems with food and other substances, are GPs doing enough? Surely she should have offered some sort of counselling (or shown some sort of interest).

'I am aware you can get slimming classes and gym membership on the NHS. At 18 stone 4, surely I would qualify for that, yet never have I been offered it or has it even been mentioned. Surely prevention is better than cure!'

'I went for my ultrasound scan when I was pregnant,' wrote Monica S, 'and the technician told me that I might not see my baby at all because the machine might not be able to see through so much fat. I was devastated. I should have walked out, but all I wanted was to see my baby, so I put up with the humiliation of climbing on to the bed and hearing her huff and puff with exasperation as she tried to get a picture. But I don't think she was really trying – she'd given up on me as soon as I walked in the door. In the end she said, "Well, you'll just have to make do with hearing the heartbeat." What should have been a magical moment was utterly ruined by her careless attitude. One day I'm going to have the courage to go back and complain. But when you are fat, you don't, because you feel as though everything is your fault.'

Fat is funny

That's right, fat is funny – until you are fat yourself. Fat has been used for comedy since ancient times. Comedians have often used fat as a rich source of mirth. One famous American comedian, George Carlin, defended his stance in his autobiographical book, *Brain Droppings*:

I used the word fat. I used that word because that's what fat people are. They're fat. They're not large; they're not stout, chunky, hefty, or plump. And they're not big-boned. Dinosaurs are big-boned. These people are not necessarily obese, either. Obese is a medical term. And they're not overweight. Overweight implies there is some correct weight. There is no correct weight. Heavy is also a misleading term. An aircraft carrier is heavy; it's not fat. Only people are fat, and that's what fat people are. They're fat. I offer no apologies for this. It is not intended as a criticism or insult. It is simply descriptive language. I don't like euphemisms. Euphemisms are a form of lying. Fat people are not gravitationally disadvantaged. They're fat. I prefer seeing things the way they are, not the way some people wish they were...

JUST A LAUGH?

Q   What do you call two fat men having a chat?

A   A heavy discussion.

✳   I wouldn't say you're fat, but you have more chins than a Hong Kong telephone directory.

✳   Inside every fat person is a thin person crying to get out – but you can usually shut them up with biscuits.

✳   She looked as if she had been poured into her clothes and had forgotten to say 'when'.

✳   Shame to hear about the choirboy from *Britain's Got Talent* being bullied. But it's something many talent-show kids have to live with. I remember hearing about the time the school bully stole Michelle McManus's dinner money and bought himself a Ford Escort.

Q   Why does everyone love Americans?

A   Thanks to them we're not the fattest nation in the world.

Monica: [looking at old home video in *Friends*] I wasn't that fat. The camera adds ten pounds!
Chandler: Just how many cameras are on you?

Of course, there have always been fat jokes – and fat jokers. The idea of the stupid fattie was very popular in children's literature – in fact, it still is. You can possibly excuse the *Magnet* comic way back in 1908 for featuring a fat kid called Billy Bunter, who was always stealing cakes and nicking his schoolmates' sweets. Then, the fat boy was a figure of fun, not a symptom of an obesity epidemic that's engulfing our primary schools. (In fact, Billy Bunter would be 100 now if he'd lived. But, as many fans pointed out in the year of his centenary, he'd probably have died long ago from heart disease, type 2 diabetes, stroke, cancer or gout.)

But can we excuse the fact that fat kids are still used as figures of fun, scorn, abuse and ridicule in modern kids' literature? Just look at the Harry Potter stories. Harry's cousin, Dudley Dursley – very much the hate figure – is spoilt, pampered and...*fat*.

'Dudley was very fat and hated exercise, unless of course it involved punching somebody. His favourite punch-bag was Harry, but he didn't often catch him. Harry didn't look it, but he was very fast. Dudley was so large his bottom drooped over the side of the kitchen chair,' wrote J.K. Rowling in the first book, *Harry Potter and the Philosopher's Stone*. Rowling took a lot of stick for that, particularly as she has publicly complained about the way we in Britain are body-obsessed and driving teenage girls to anorexia. But authors like her should understand, according to a top professor of children's literature, that they're part of that very problem.

'Dudley is a fat little rotter and his obesity is presented as a moral failing,' says Professor Jean Webb of Worcester University.

'For years and years we have all been conditioned through the culture of fat kids being reviled in children's books. They're demonising overweight kids by portraying fat characters as spoilt, greedy and mean. In fact, by making weight an issue at all, they're just contributing to the distorted values about body image in society.'

Professor Webb reckons that kids' literature over the past 100 years paints the evolution of the imperialist boy hero – athletic, slim and handsome – the epitome of masculinity. This, she says, has marginalised and effeminised the fat child.

And where does the fault lie? 'I trace it back to the Church,' she replies, 'the portrayal of gluttony as a vice, as immoral. Contrast that with the emergence of the muscular Christian ideal and you have the roots of fat prejudice.

'Just look at Billy Bunter,' continues Professor Webb, who's now part of a growing academic 'taskforce' trying to question and challenge prevailing attitudes about children and obesity. 'He's fat, obviously. But there's something stupidly effeminate about his coiffured hair. And the lustful, lascivious way he crams buns into his mouth – well, there's a sexuality to it that is designed to debase his character.

'Piggy in *Lord of the Flies* is the character most victimised – because he's fat, asthmatic, wears thick Billy Bunter-style glasses and is seen by the other boys as pathetic. He can't do anything for himself and constantly tries to get out of work. Ultimately, Piggy can't even save himself from his fate.'

New authors, though, are beginning to challenge this old-fashioned attitude. Jean Webb wants more children's authors to challenge the preconceptions rife in so much of children's literature.

'Wouldn't it be great to see a tubby hero, for a change? Or, better still, great writing that doesn't deem a child's size to be a sign of character?'

Showbiz stereotyping

Can you ever get on in show business or the theatre if you're fat? Clearly you can if your talent shines brightly and hugely enough to eclipse your girth. In fact, there are quite a few glowing examples in the world of comedy and music. But it's not so easy if you are a new talent – someone trying to compete for your debut in the limelight. Look at *Pop Idol* near-winner Rik Waller, who is probably remembered as much for his size as for his impressive singing voice. (The British media saw to that. The *Sun* called him 'The 22-year-old man mountain', 'the 30st giant whose weight and looks were overshadowed by his fabulous voice' and the 'roly-poly *Pop Idol* star'.)

Simon Cowell was widely reported as saying that Rik only got down to the last few on the *Pop Idol* programme because 'he was fat', and that he couldn't win because he was 'too fat to be an idol'. Perhaps true, but interestingly, Cowell had to see past the fat for the second series, and so too did the voting audience, when Michelle McManus (5 feet 2 inches and 20 stone) won with a terrific singing voice but a body more traditionally suited to opera!

However, even the world of opera has modernised its view towards obesity. Now that Luciano Pavarotti is dead, it seems that opera directors feel able to acknowledge the elephant in the room – the obesity of some of their hugest talents.

Time was when an obese diva soprano was worshipped and adored, even if it stretched the audience's imagination that a 25-stone prima donna could be the romantic heroine dying of consumption. Audiences were used to suspending disbelief. One of the most famous coloratura sopranos from the 1930s was the Rubenesque Luisa Tetrazzini, who had a spaghetti dish named after her. It is said she could barely fit inside her dressing room. But no one questioned it.

The magnificent Jessye Norman, who they said 'cut an impressive, enormous figure before her audiences', once sued a music magazine for calling her fat. 'At Covent Garden,' said one review, 'she statuesquely sang the title role of Strauss's *Ariadne auf Naxos*. At the close, she embraced the stick-thin tenor James King into the folds of her majestic, tent-like garment, from which he was never seen to emerge.'

But welcome to the 21st century – because when diva Deborah Voigt was hired to sing the same role at London's Royal Opera House in Covent Garden, she was fired for being fat. It caused outright shock and horror in the world of opera. Never before had a female singer been too fat!

Real life

'I was terribly distressed and angry,' she said. 'But part of me understood. I have always wanted to sing the role of Salome – but I would have had to reinterpret the sexy "Dance of the Seven Veils" as the "Dance of the 77 Veils"! So I did always want to lose weight.'

That summer, she got herself a gastric bypass operation – and has now lost 15 stone. At a trim size 14, she returned to the Covent Garden stage in June 2008, singing the part from which she was sacked.

'Perhaps the cruelty did kick-start me into something I should have done years ago,' she says now. 'But I was never fat because I was lazy or stupid – I was addicted to food. I used food the way that alcoholics use alcohol and drug addicts use drugs. If I was sad, I ate; if I was happy, I ate; if I was lonely, I ate. And I grew up sitting on a piano stool and singing and not running around playing soccer. Only my fingers were in great shape.'

Peter Katona, the casting director who fired Voigt, was quoted in a Sunday newspaper as saying that opera singers often used the myth that fat people had more powerful voices as an 'excuse' to eat too much. 'They say, "In order to be able to sing well, I need to eat a lot",' he claimed. 'Well, it's not true.'

You have to be careful what you say, even in the world of pop. One group actually walked out of a *Top of the Pops* recording after an ill-judged introduction from Richard Bacon, the presenter. He said something about 'a big, fat melting pot', and the Magic Numbers decided that was one jibe too many. They're a family band – two brothers and two sisters – and they're not particularly large, but they are proud of being natural. They issued a statement: 'Due to derogatory, unfunny remarks made during the guest presenter's introduction to our performance, we felt we had to make a stand and leave. It was an important day for us and should have been special. We didn't take this decision lightly but we stand by it.' Bacon protested that he didn't mean it like that.

Peter Stringfellow also 'didn't mean it like that' when he allegedly banned fat people from his nightclub. Apparently some woman had turned up not looking like Kylie Minogue, and he'd told his bouncers to stop her coming in, even though she was with lots of nice-looking slim girls. He was reported to have commented: 'What's the point in going to a nice place if it's not surrounded by nice people that you want to look at?'

And his 'operations manager' apparently added: 'The majority of fat people have great difficulty in dressing appropriately. They don't take as much care with their appearance as slim people. Invariably, that means fat sloppy people are refused access to the club.'

Stringfellow later explained: 'This woman walked in and she was a terrible mess. She was really big, but not only that, she was sloppy with it. She was wearing flat shoes and was shuffling around. I said to my manager, "Who the hell is that?" and he explained she was with a group of gorgeous girls. I said, "I don't care, she can't be in here." ...a day later it was all over the front page of the *Sun* and went round the world. People were outside with placards. I had calls from Australia, Japan – from all over. I felt stupid and I had to do some pretty major backtracking.' (McGibbon 2006)

We're all prejudiced

Thoughtless comments betray a serious fat prejudice inside all of us. Fat prejudice bolsters public ridicule and insulting, ignorant stereotypes in the media. Fat people can legally be discriminated against in virtually every country in the world. Fat people are blamed for their own problems, and are treated with contempt. According to one size acceptance group: 'Our culture has the idea that fat people are somehow less than human, and therefore shouldn't share the simple human right of fair and decent treatment.'

Being fat doesn't give just *you* a hard time either. It rubs off on your partner and friends too. A group of obesity researchers at Liverpool University found hard evidence that society doesn't stigmatise only the fattie – people also make judgements about their friends and families.

The researchers showed a cross-section of people two photographs – one of a man and his fat partner, the other of the same man with a slim partner. There was a huge difference in the way he was perceived. People liked him when he had a slim wife, but abhorred him – said he was less trustworthy, miserable, self-indulgent, passive, shapeless, depressed, weak, unattractive, insignificant and insecure – when he was married to an obese woman.

Dr Jason Halford, who led the research, said in an interview with BBC Online, 'This showed his personality is being judged on *her* physical characteristics. It proves the extent of obesity stigmatisation. We should raise awareness of obesity discrimination.'

It all seems to confirm the old nursery rhyme: 'Fatty and Skinny went to bed; Fatty rolled over and Skinny was dead.' Perhaps the prejudice starts at nursery rhyme age.

Yet more studies – in Canada – show that fat prejudice is rife among kids. Show kindergarten-age children silhouettes of an obese child and they apparently describe them as 'lazy, dirty, stupid, ugly, cheats and liars'.

Show children and adults simple black-and-white line drawings of a normal-weight child, an obese child, and children with various handicaps, including missing hands and facial disfigurement, and both children and adults rate the obese child as the least likeable. This prejudice extends across races, across rural and urban dwellers, and, saddest of all, even to obese persons themselves.

Mary Portas, who presents *Mary Queen of Shops* on TV, agrees. Her role is to go into failing businesses, identify where they're going wrong, and put it right. In one programme she was troubleshooting a boutique that ostensibly catered for the larger woman, and she quickly decided that it was 'fattist' attitudes that were the root of the problem. The shop was being run by a woman who, subconsciously, showed contempt for the very women she wanted to be her clients. She held up the most awful tent of a dress and proudly proclaimed that this was 'for the no-hopers', that it would cover up all bumps and bulges, and fit the woman who was too fat for anything nice. She referred to her clients as 'bouncy castles' or 'bullets' or having 'funny necks'.

Mary reckoned she was trying to sell clothes that most people, whatever their size, wouldn't be seen dead in. Mary reminded her that 57 per cent of British women were over size 14 – and they all had a right to look fabulous.

Yet more university researchers – at the University of British Columbia in Canada – seem to have found a scientific reason for prejudice against fat. Apparently, we're programmed to view the obese as a health threat.

The research, reported in the journal *Evolution and Human Behaviour*, claims that our brains have evolved to react to excessive body fat as an outward sign of disease. This is the way we see rashes and inflammations. It's important that we instinctively know they're bad because the bacteria and viruses that cause them are invisible. Similarly, we heave at the mere sight of rotting food. It's a defensive mechanism.

'Antipathy towards obese people is a powerful and pervasive prejudice in many contemporary populations,' said the team from the University of British Columbia. 'So thin people instinctively dislike fat people because their immune system associates fat with infection and sends out a signal of disgust – it's a Darwinian response.'

Darwinian it may be, but I reckon it's no excuse for prejudice in a modern world. Fat people are human beings, and they hurt when patronised, pilloried or even pitied.

'Why is there so much hostility?' wailed one buddy on my website recently. 'Why can't they get at people who are truly corrupt and dishonest and mean, not ordinary people like me who are trying the best they can to hold their heads up in a world that's trying its damnedest to drown them?'

Louise Diss, who used to run TOAST (The Obesity Awareness and Solutions Trust), tells lots of dreadful yet funny stories about weight prejudice. She herself lost 10 stone, so she knows what it's like to be obese.

'I remember going out to lunch with a group of girlfriends,' she says. 'I was the only fattie, the others were fairly slim, but we had all had a good main course. Then came time for desserts. Only one girl ordered something – a big slice of cheesecake. The rest of us just settled for coffee. The waitress took the order and disappeared. Minutes later, a different waitress brought the cheesecake. Not knowing who had ordered it, she simply assumed, and delivered it straight to me! She brought it to me because I was the fat one. It was an assumption that spoke volumes about our innate prejudice and judgemental attitude to fat. And it broke my heart at the time.'

Another story she tells in horror is of the newspaper that reported a case of sexual abuse. The headline said: '24 Stone Paedophile Sent to Prison'.

'Isn't it unbelievable that his weight gets the first mention,' remarks Louise, 'as though his weight is much more offensive than the fact that he is a paedophile?'

'When a thin person looks at a fat person, the thin person considers the fat person less virtuous than he,' writes Judith Moore in her memoir, *Fat Girl*. 'The fat person lacks willpower, pride, this wretched attitude "self-esteem", and does not care about friends and family because if he or she did care about friends and family, he or she would not wander the Earth looking like a repulsive sow, rhinoceros, hippo, elephant, general wide-mawed, flesh-flopping, flabby monster.'

There's something else weird about society's scorn for the obese. They're reviled for their size, but they're also reviled for their attempts to lose weight. Only when they have successfully lost weight and can show off a trim figure do they gain society's acceptance. But woe betide them if they ever slip up. Human fallibility is no excuse.

Candida Crewe, who wrote a compelling book, *Eating Myself*, about her lifelong battle with body image and weight, says fat people rarely enjoy food. They see it only as a guilty pleasure.

She is particularly strong on what she calls 'fattism' – the last permissible prejudice.

❬❬ We frown upon homophobia, sexism and all the rest, but wince with disdain as a member of the super-sized community waddles and wheezes past. Once they are safely out of earshot we might even use unkind terms, such as 'lard arse'. ❭❭

Her memoir chronicles her fight against what she thought was overweight – in fact, she never was. She tormented herself needlessly for years. But it all taught her so much about society and how our kids' minds can be warped by crazy values about food, weight and prejudice. Crewe castigates the fashion industry for favouring models 'who resemble spaghetti, but never eat it'. She speculates that women are tempted to diet because they find it easier to go without food than men do: in times of need down the centuries, women starved themselves so their children and husbands could eat.

In a very famous and groundbreaking article in the American *Ladies' Home Journal* back in the 1990s, writer Leslie Lampert reported that she had donned a fat suit for a week and how shocked she was by society's hatred of fat people.

'Mostly, I became angry,' she told me. 'Angry because what I experienced in the week that I wore that fat suit, designed to make me look like a 250 plus-pound woman, was that our society not only hates fat people, it feels entitled to participate in a prejudice that at many levels parallels racism and religious bigotry. And in a country that prides itself on being sensitive to the handicapped and the homeless, the obese continue to be the target of cultural abuse.

'I got the idea after watching Goldie Hawn wear a fat suit for *Death Becomes Her.* I thought, I wonder what it would really be like to look so big? Then I asked myself, what would it be like to live like that? I read about some former fat people (all of whom had lost significant amounts of weight after intestinal bypass surgery), who said they'd rather be blind, deaf or have a leg amputated than be fat again. I thought – can it really be that bad?

'So every day for a week I put on 200 lb [14 stone]. My kids looked scared of me. My husband held back. I found it really difficult even to sleep. I became depressed, self-conscious and miserable very quickly – and paranoid about food. When it was all over and I could take that suit off, I didn't feel elated – just sad. I felt ashamed of my culture and how much pain we cause people who are less than our concept of ideal.'

Where America leads…

Such cruelty is not just inhuman – it can make it almost impossible to help fat people help themselves. That's the view of one of Australia's leading obesity experts, Professor John Dixon, who is part of the country's leading anti-obesity task force. You wouldn't think that such a country, synonymous with the great outdoors, surfing, sport and seafood, would have an obesity problem at all, but in fact Australia is only just behind the USA in the obesity stakes. Nearly half of its women and two-thirds of its men are overweight or obese.

According to some reports, Australia officially became the fattest nation on Earth in the summer of 2008. Aussie obesity specialists deny this, but acknowledge that it's already more 'normal' to have a weight problem Down Under than not. And they're worried because obesity is spreading fast in their children. Ghastly predictions reckon that by 2010 some 70 per cent of Australians will be above their healthy weight range.

Against that backdrop, you'd expect them to be proactively search-ing for an answer. 'Yet we still stigmatise the obese,' Professor Dixon told me. 'By the time people get to see me, they have already been so damaged by society's attitudes that they are almost impos-sible to help... They say things like: "I am so stupid, I can't lose weight. I fail every diet I've ever tried. I'm just a big fat lazy pig."

'They blame themselves because society already blames them, and therefore society must be right. They are cruel to themselves because that's their norm. No one has ever been compassionate to them – no one's ever cared. All they've had is abuse and ridicule. I wonder how I am ever to help them take charge of their lifestyles and turn their lives around if they hate themselves so much.

'Yet I believe these patients are suffering from an addiction. They are addicted to food – they crave it, and they have no off switch to tell them they've had enough. On top of that, they live in a society that promotes food and eating as entertainment and a leisure pursuit. Yet that same society persecutes them for getting fat on it. They can't help getting fat on it. It's a compulsion.'

Another top obesity expert in Philadelphia sums it up: 'We live in a society that largely scorns obesity and overvalues thinness.' These are the words of Gary D. Foster, PhD, who is clinical direc-tor of the weight and eating disorders programme at the Univer-sity of Pennsylvania School of Medicine in Philadelphia. He spe-cialises in helping obese patients who've failed most weight-loss programmes – and his success record is high.

'People often say things like, "I cheated today on my diet",' Fos-ter says. 'What does that mean, "cheated"? How would you feel if your teenage son or daughter came home and said they got caught cheating on a test, or, worse yet, your spouse came home and said, "I got caught cheating at work today"? How did a bag of M&Ms ever get equated with something like cheating?'

Blaming people who are obese for being obese is like blaming someone who has a cold for having a cold – it doesn't help. Instead of making people guilty about their weight, says Foster, doctors must help patients to learn what they need to know to gain control of their eating habits and behaviours related to food.

❦❦ *Losing weight is about skills not wills.* ❦❦

'We say this to patients a lot: it's about skills, not wills. I don't think that people who go on a diet lack will-power; it's just that they lack skills to eat less and move more in a society that teaches them to do just the opposite. It's just a different skill set, much like learning to play the piano or driving a car.'

Fatties get sidelined

A final sad fact is that if you're fat, you'll miss out on your proper place in history.

How many queens have we had in the UK – proper queens who have reigned in their own name? Victoria, of course. The two Elizabeths, I can hear you say. And Mary Tudor. But how many of you remember Anne (1702–14)? The last of the Stuarts.

Robert Bucholz, a history professor at Loyola University in Chicago, has spent years trying to figure out why Queen Anne, who was an important British monarch, has had so little attention. Apart from antique experts often praising the shape of 'Queen Anne legs' on *Antiques Roadshow*, she never gets a mention – not even in history books.

'Few people even think about her,' says Bucholz. Finally, he figured out why: she was fat. Now he feels so strongly about it that he lectures on the way such prejudice can alter history.

He told me: 'In recent years, Queen Anne has been recognised by historians of her period as a highly effective monarch who defeated the most powerful ruler of her day, Louis XIV; skilfully balanced the power between two powerful political parties (the Whigs and the Tories); presided over a period of relative prosperity; all with a minimum of constitutional chicanery or terror. (There was but one execution for high treason in her reign.) It could be argued that she was Britain's first truly successful constitutional monarch (post-1688) and that she set the pattern in this regard for her successors. Elizabeth I could not say so much, yet the book and video shelves groan with accounts of her life, while Anne goes neglected.'

Why? Could it really have been an image problem due to her weight? The professor is sure of it!

'One reason was Anne's quiet personality and tendency to delegate. But another, I am sure, was her weight. We do not know how much Anne weighed, but she has always been recognised as a fat woman. Contemporaries danced around this when she was queen, but posthumous commentators have generally seen it as an index of her abilities. That is, almost *invariably*, historians who dwell upon her obesity regard her as weak, incompetent, easily led. Historians who minimise her weight or ignore it tend to think that she was a pretty good queen!'

Bucholz isn't alone in this conclusion. Another historian at Harvard has acknowledged both Anne's girth and her greatness.

It seems to me that this connects with a number of much larger issues. First, aren't historians supposed to be objective? Just what does Anne's size have to do with her abilities?

'Historians work within their own time,' says Bucholz, 'and... when was the last time you heard the words "fat" and "competent" or "obese" and "effective" in the same sentence? Yet the world is surely filled with fat, obese people of ability and accomplishment.

What is wrong with us that we cannot seem to hold the two to-gether in our minds?

❝ This is not an argument for being fat or gaining weight as positive things in and of themselves. The health issues are too significant. It is an argument for taking fat people as people, relegating their appear-ance and size to the category "irrelevant" when it comes to ability or accomplishment. **❞**

I point out that one of our greatest queens, Victoria, was stout.

'Ah, yes!' agrees Professor Bucholz. 'She did eventually grow stout – not surprising given the number of pregnancies – but this may have been a positive advantage in conveying a maternal image. It is only in *our* day that Victoria has become a slightly ridiculous figure. We are merciless: witness the tabloid and late-night comic treatment of Al Gore, Cherie Blair, Bill Clinton, Hillary Clinton, etc. All people of ability; all attacked rather easily, if irrelevantly, on the issue of weight.'

Politicians beware. Churchill might have been able to carry off being overweight while also being 'fattist' – according to one fa-mous story, a woman told Churchill: 'You are drunk, Sir Winston, you are disgustingly drunk'. To which he replied: 'Yes, Mrs Brad-dock, I am drunk. But you, Mrs Braddock, are ugly and disgust-ingly fat. Tomorrow morning, though, I, Winston Churchill, will be sober. But you, Mrs Braddock, will still be ugly and fat.' – but nowadays a fat politician, like Churchill's great-grandson, Nicho-las Soames MP, might find it more difficult to be taken seriously and treated respectfully. Soames has been called a 'one-man food mountain' and nicknamed 'Fat Boy Dim' by the *Sunday Times*.

Back to Queen Anne. As Professor Bucholz told me her story, I started to feel terribly sad for her. By 1700, Anne had been pregnant at least 18 times, and 13 times she miscarried or gave birth to stillborn children. Of the remaining five children, four died before reaching the age of two years. Her only son to survive infancy, William, Duke of Gloucester, died at the age of 11 on 29 July 1700. To add to her troubles, she was addicted to brandy and nicknamed Brandy Nan. No wonder she was fat. She was stressed, unhappy, her body racked by so many pregnancies, no children to love and a dead husband. She died of an abscess and fever arising from gout on 1 August 1714. Her body was so swollen that it had to be buried in Westminster Abbey in a vast, almost-square coffin.

Poor woman! Please let's not remember her for being fat. Sadly, though, the most famous portrait of her shows a very dour, unhappy-looking woman, her large body squeezed into a tightly corseted dress. Ironically, ratcheting yourself into a corset is supposed to be one of the new, 21st-century ways of losing weight and staying slim: it holds you in so tight, you can barely breathe, let alone eat. I've tried one and I have to say – it works! However, you do end up with a strained expression like poor Queen Anne's.

CHAPTER 2

APPEARANCES CAN BE DECEPTIVE

✳

A s I've complained before, we live in a society that's obsessed with the superficial image – the outside of our body. But I have news for you. Thin people can be fat on the inside. And they're a growing species! What's more, their fat could be much more dangerous than the stuff that's wobbling around on your thighs and bum (more of that later).

OK, if you are hugely overweight, it's likely you are unhealthy through and through, I'm afraid. But it has also now been proved that some fat people are healthier than some thin ones – not just because they may be fit and do lots of exercise, but because they have more of the better sort of fat.

There are two sorts of fat, you see.

Subcutaneous fat lies just under the skin. On some obese people it can be several inches thick. But it's relatively harmless in itself. It disappears pretty sharpish when a patient diets.

Visceral fat lies deeper inside the body, often wrapped around and marbled through the vital organs. It's much harder to shift, and it's the most dangerous type. Its existence seems to be linked with conditions such as diabetes and heart disease, and the only way to get rid of it is through exercise.

The more subcutaneous fat you have, the more visceral fat you'll get. However, deposits of these fats around the body depend not just on what you eat, but on your genes too.

Genes are also the reason why some people get fat and others don't. Experts all over the world are finding that some races are predisposed to visceral fat. Asian men particularly put weight on around the middle but not so much on their bums and legs. This 'apple' shape usually means large amounts of visceral fat wrapped around and marbled through vital organs. Genetically, Afro-Caribbean people tend to get fat in a 'pear-shaped' way. They might weigh more than 'apples', but could have the less dangerous sort of fat. Similarly, men seem to put weight on differently than women, so there is a hormonal element to the disposition of fat.

Even within the same gender and race there can be variations in how the body deals with fat. While one cube of chocolate goes straight to my hips, I have friends who seem to snack all day and can still shimmy into the flimsiest of summer dresses and boast about their size 10 jeans. One of my best mates runs an ice-cream company in rural Devon, and she's slurping her own creations all day – in the interests of designing new flavours. You should see the cream and sugar that goes into her work – and then into her mouth! Yet at 50+ she can fit into all her daughter's clothes – they're both slim. Daughter is, as you'd expect, very active. But my mate isn't. Over the years, she has watched me in my battle against weight, from behind her copy of *Heat* magazine and packet of Maryland cookies. She has seen me slaving away in the gym or madly doing aerobics in front of the TV just to try and lose a dress size for summer – and she sits and scoffs.

She's one of those people you hate shopping with. You know, she's trying on a size 12 jacket that you couldn't possibly stretch around your arms and she stands in front of the mirror, whining:

'I don't know why you couldn't fit this one, pet – it's absolutely huge on me.'

She can't understand, and neither can I, why we both started out at the beginning of our friendship – 25 years ago – as trim and tiny, yet I have ended up with a weight problem and she hasn't. Well, scientists have been working on that conundrum for years, and they're getting nearer and nearer to the answer. And although it won't necessarily help me to lose weight and keep it off, it does represent a giant slap in the face of the Snotty Self-Righteous who delight in remarks like:

'Slimming isn't rocket science, you know!'
'Just do some exercise and stop eating chips.'
'I eat healthily and I have never had a problem.'
'Don't you have any will-power?'

These people, so smug in their slimness, are in for a shock. Let's look at what the latest research reveals.

Hidden horrors

No one ever mentions that when you get fat, you put weight on your insides too. Why hasn't anyone ever made a big deal of it? Doctors say they've always known, but I reckon most people are unaware.

You know how exhausting it can be to walk home from the shop with several large carriers, or maybe a bag of potatoes or a couple of cans of paint? Just a simple walk from the supermarket to the car park can get you all stressed out, sweaty or panting? Yet those few kilograms are a tiny proportion of the extra weight you probably carry around as fat all the time.

A big bag of King Edwards is 2.5 kg; a 5-litre can of paint is 7 kg. Carry a can in each hand and try walking far without moaning – and yet that's just an extra 1½ stone! Even if you weren't puffing and blowing, the muscles in your arms would certainly feel the strain. If, like I was a year ago, you're 4 stone overweight, you are effectively carrying around three times that paint burden day in, day out. It's even weighing down on you while you sleep.

Now imagine that the muscles and organs inside your body are similarly weighed down. Important muscles, such as your heart, and organs such as liver, kidneys and lungs. Fat settles on your waist, hips, thighs and bum in a thick layer, but when it's deposited around your inside organs, it is marbled through them too – like the sort of steak you would refuse at a posh restaurant.

Tiny particles of fat also swim along in your bloodstream, looking for places to settle. In fact, an obese body can hide a dismal interior, full of potential problems. It's rather like the sort of 'challenge property' they feature on TV's *Homes Under the Hammer,* where presenter Martin Roberts dons his hard hat, shakes his head knowingly and tells viewers: 'Well, this house looks derelict from the outside, but just wait till you go in!' And then there's a horror combination of dry rot, damp rot, warped floorboards and fire damage that is going to bankrupt you.

One American surgeon spelt it out frankly on TV in *Living Large in America: Inside the Body.* Dr Nancy Snyderman even cut through a huge side of fatty beef to demonstrate. Inside an obese body, she said, this is what you'll find:

'First, the heart is probably enlarged because it has grown bigger, enabling it to work so much harder to pump blood around a bigger than average body. In fact, for each 2.2 lb of fat a body gains, the body must create 2 miles of blood vessels to feed the extra mass.

'The liver would also have grown to nearly twice its normal size, but instead of a reddish-brown colour, it would likely be a greasy yellow – caused by residue from the extra fat that encases it. The lungs, however, would be smaller than normal, crushed underneath all that extra body mass they'd be forced to support. This would make breathing harder.

'Obesity can make it extra difficult for a doctor to diagnose any patient because he has to see past (or through) the layers of fat in X-rays. In an operating theatre, obesity makes operating time longer, surgeons have to make a bigger incision, they have to move the retractors around a lot more, it takes longer to close the wound – it all adds up to extra risk.

'Surgeons have to cut through inches and inches of fat – this is hard work, slows down the process and the fat makes your hands slippery. The bigger the incision, the more needs to heal – risk of infection is higher...there's a longer recovery time...

'If you're fatter, you are going to need more medicine because you are a bigger person, and a lot of the anaesthesia drugs linger in the fat, they're fat soluble, they don't wash out of your body so quickly, so not only are you going to get more drug, you're going to be more hung over, you'll feel lousier longer!

'When you go up a step, you are putting pressure seven times your body weight on your knee joints, so an obese person's knees are at increased risk for injury with each and every pound.

'There's a risk to doctors too in dealing with obese patients – just typical injuries in trying to move the patients. Increasingly, we are waking people up earlier to ask them to move themselves because nursing staff do not want to break their backs.'

Then she put it succinctly, with a motoring metaphor clearly intended to appeal to men: 'When we're born, we're like neat little pick-up trucks, all shiny and new. But when you become obese, you go from being that neat little pick-up truck to a heavy-load dumper truck carrying far too much, and your axle will bust. Everything will be affected, your knees, ankles, hips – everything internally too will give in. You're a mess.' (Snyderman 2007)

Thanks for the subtlety, Nancy, but we get the point. Fat isn't just about what's on the outside. Inside, fatter organs may be struggling to do their jobs.

I was enthusing about my new-found knowledge to Dr David Bull, who often sits next to me on TV's *The Wright Stuff*. He had more to offer:

'Even your veins and arteries get thicker, so the space for the blood to flow is restricted. Not only does this change the speed, it actually changes the way your blood flows through the vein – like whooshing in a spiral, knocking against the vessel walls, knocking off bits of fatty deposit that can then cause obstruction...'

Sounds even more dangerous than *Fantastic Voyage* (Donald Pleasence, Raquel Welch, 1966), where they miniaturised a submarine and crew and injected them into a man's bloodstream to break up a blood clot in his brain. If you haven't seen it, you can just imagine the problems they encountered – without the extra difficulty of an obese patient!

Right, that's the bottom line. Fat on the inside endangers your heart, liver, lungs, kidneys and even your blood. But, until recently, who knew that it could happen to skinny people? Pathologists knew it. Over the years they became accustomed to seeing that apparently slim people could have large quantities of fat deep inside them and marbled through vital organs.

Now we know that fat is a double-edged sword, but how can we tell the extent of the two types in our body?

Ways of measuring fat

Surely we can tell if we're fat by just looking in a mirror? Do we need scales, charts and calculations to tell us if we're overweight, obese, or morbidly obese? Well, some people seem to think so, but the latest research shows that they could be putting their faith in the wrong thing.

Body mass index

Every obesity specialist I've met throughout the world now reckons that BMI (body mass index – a calculation of your weight versus your height) is a very poor way of measuring whether someone is fat, obese or morbidly obese. We now know that an Olympic athlete whose body is heavy with hardened muscle can have the same BMI as an unfit man or woman with 4 or 5 stone of fat. It also means that a plump lady who exercises regularly could have a higher BMI than a less rounded woman who sits in a chair all day. So it is no measure of health!

❝ Sumo wrestlers eat up to 5000 calories a day and have a BMI of 56, yet they have very little internal fat. They have low cholesterol, low insulin resistance and a low level of fatty acids. Their fat is all stored under the skin, not around their organs, so they're surprisingly healthy. ❞

WHAT'S YOUR BMI?

Body mass index, or BMI, is the number you get when you divide your weight in kilograms by your height in centimetres squared. I know – who thought of that, for heaven's sake? (Apparently, it was dreamed up in the 1850s by a Belgian social scientist called Adolphe Quetelet...

You didn't really need to know that, did you?) Given what we now know about the different types of fat and where they are deposited around the body, BMI is a pretty unscientific way of measuring it. Nonetheless, if you want to know how the calculation is made, here it is...

First, get hold of a set of scales that weighs in kilos, a tape measure marked in centimetres and a calculator. It's also helpful to have a son or daughter on hand who's at least year 8 in maths! (Failing these things, go to one of the many websites where there's a simple and instant calculator that'll do the job for you!)

Now, let's say you're a woman who's 5 feet 5 inches (1.65 metres) and 12 stone (76 kg).

* Multiply your height by itself: 1.65 x 1.65 = 2.72
* Divide your weight by the figure you've just calculated: 76 ÷ 2.72 = 27.9

This means your BMI is 28. Check your result against the list below and you'll see you're overweight but not yet obese.

Less than 18.5 Underweight (you might need to gain weight for your health's sake)

18.5–24.9 Normal range

25–29.9 Overweight (you might want to lose some weight for your health's sake, or at least prevent further weight gain)

30–35 Obese (your health is at risk)

Over 35 Very obese (you should visit your doctor for a health check, as you might need extra help to manage your weight and health. This is especially important before taking up any new exercise.)

Over 40 Morbidly obese (you could develop other problems or co-morbidities caused by your obesity)

The trouble with BMI is that it doesn't take into account the fact that muscle weighs so much more than fat. This means that the BMI formula makes it possible for a healthy, muscular athlete with very low body fat to be classified as obese. BMI also tells you nothing about where your fat is deposited, whether your fat is visceral (the harmful kind around and within your internal organs) or adipose (all over your bum and thighs). That's why many doctors and health organisations are advising people to pay more attention to their waist measurement – because that clearly indicates whether you're an apple or a pear, the former being rather more at risk than the latter.

To measure your waist accurately, hold a tape measure around your middle at belly button level. Note the number, then check the information below:

WOMEN
32–35 in (81–88 cm) carries a risk similar to a BMI of 25–30.
More than 35 in (88 cm) carries a risk similar to a BMI greater than 30.

MEN
37–40 in (94–102 cm) carries a risk similar to a BMI of 25–30.
More than 40 in (102 cm) carries a risk similar to a BMI greater than 30.

It sounds quaint, but if your trousers or skirt feel too tight around the middle, that's the time to check your waist.

Source: all figures from the National Obesity Forum

The thing is, we all want to quantify problems, and fat is no exception. But by looking for a 'diagnosis', aren't we over-medicalising? Aren't we just allowing ourselves to be blinded by science in order to shy away from the true facts – that we're fat and we know it? Well, not entirely. Not when people like Marie Parker (see page 45) are refused a job on the basis of BMI alone. Not when insurance companies demand some proof of your fitness and health, or they refuse to insure you. Not when you can be refused an operation – like a hip replacement – because of your high BMI figure. Not while blame is still such a big part of the obesity debate.

Looking in a mirror will tell you whether or not you like your own shape. Shopping for clothes will immediately give you an idea of your size, in retail terms. Trying to buckle up your seatbelt in an aeroplane will give you an idea of your girth. And listening to the taunts of children on the bus may convince you of your less-than-perfect body image. But none of that says anything about your health and fitness.

So scientists are indeed working on new ideas to tell you about the fat on your body, how it is distributed, and particularly whether or not you have too much of the toxic kind, the visceral fat – the stuff that could be lurking around your vital organs, or clogging up your arteries.

I took the plunge and decided to try out a couple of these new diagnostic machines myself. And both experiences convinced me that I must get a grip on my daily routine so that I can do more exercise. And on my food intake, which is still too snacky, with too many unconscious calories.

Body volume index

Dr Asad Rahim, who's the lead physician for obesity services at one of the Midlands' top hospitals, uses a special type of scanner –

basically a very posh 3-D camera – to take an all-round picture of the body. This body volume index (BVI) scan shows precisely where the fat is lying and will, he hopes, help motivate people towards their goal of losing weight. He strongly believes that it's a lot more help than giving them their BMI.

Sadly – and fascinatingly – the evidence to date shows that not even a 3-D picture of your own fat body *does* help with motivation. So far, it doesn't seem to be making any difference as to whether someone becomes more determined to reach their slimming and fitness goal. But it does help the doctors figure out why you're fat, whether you have too much of the dangerous fat, and whereabouts all that subcutaneous stuff is lurking. And across a population the images help them to work out fat trends – whether people of certain ethnic backgrounds, gender, age, habits and so forth are prone to obesity – and can even highlight 'clusters'. Statistics seem to show clusters of obesity in Wales, though no one yet knows why.

The scanner was developed from a camera used by the retail industry to tell how we as a race are growing. Clothing firms used it to mass-produce garments in various sizes, and they soon noticed that waist, neck and torso circumferences were getting larger every year. Now it's been adapted for medical use, and we might even see scanners in health clubs soon. They look just like quick-photo booths, with the scientific clobber at one end and a black curtain at the other.

Now I haven't worn a bikini in public since I got my first job in television some 30 years ago. In fact, I remember being told – by a top TV executive – 'If you are going to stay in front of the camera, you should accept that you can never cavort half naked on a beach from now on because the photographers will always find you – anywhere in the world. And none of us,' he said, pulling in his own paunch, 'would look good in a telephoto shot spread all

over the front page of the *News of the World*.' And he was right. So
I never have.

But you have to strip down to the tighty whities for the BVI
scanner. Luckily, you can do it all totally privately, behind a black
curtain. The scanner takes about seven seconds to do its thing,
shining lights and cameras on you from all angles, in a sort of
'strobing' effect. I imagined this is what it would be like to do
a special effects shot for *The Matrix*. Then, as you fumble for
your dressing-gown and grope for your dignity, the scanner up-
loads your 3-D image to a computer for analysis. There, on the
screen, is a virtual model of you – warts and all. Cringe-making
in the extreme!

As I remarked earlier, you know how fat you are by looking in
a mirror, don't you? But here you can see it from all angles. Bird's-
eye view. Snail-on-the-pavement view. Right up close and personal.
The great thing is that there's no moral judgement. No one tut-tuts.
But they can tell, quite literally, how you are on the inside.

Me, I had a load too much subcutaneous fat in all the classic female places – around the waist, and on the hips, thighs and
posterior. In a middle-aged white female, that's pretty common. If
I'd showed a barrel-like figure, with tons of fat around my middle,
that would be more of a worry, since it would mean an overload of
visceral fat.

❝ I took my BVI picture home and stuck it on the fridge until the children complained that it put them off their food too. We all thought it
was horrendously motivational. ❞

Extra weight around the stomach and chest area is an indication
of greater health risk, and is more common in men. Particularly
Asian men. Even men who think they're quite slim.

'People of different ethnic backgrounds have a predisposition to put weight on in different regions – and that is highly relevant in diagnosing problems that are likely to develop,' says Dr Rahim. 'To give an example, the South Asian population tends to put weight on around the abdomen, and the difficulty with that is that you can be normal weight, classed by BMI, but still have a significantly increased risk of metabolic disease, such as diabetes, and that's why there's an epidemic of diabetes within the South Asian community. They may not be classed as overweight, with BMIs of 24 or 25, but they are getting weight-related disorders that could have been diagnosed and helped much earlier. It's the distribution of weight that is the key thing.'

But whatever your shape, doesn't it all come down to one thing still? How can overweight and obese people lose that fat?

Dr Rahim specialises in patients who are morbidly obese – twice their 'normal' body weight. The way obesity is growing in the Midlands, he says, means his clinics are so full that he can't get around to those who are just plain obese or overweight. Even though, research shows, they are probably going to end up at his door in a few years' time...

'The morbidly obese are actually a very small percentage of the population, about 3–4 per cent, but that's all I can concentrate on at the moment because if I started to try and help others, my clinics just couldn't cope.

'The BVI is probably more of a help to us doctors than it is to the patients. I had hoped it would help patients see a target for themselves, that it would show them progress. But so far, it hasn't helped much with motivation. For me, though, it will provide a more useful way of collating data; it'll give us better stats. We know that BMI is hopelessly inaccurate, so we're trying to develop something better. Someone can be a body builder, be pure muscle and have a BMI of 30, compared with someone who is truly obese and has a BMI of 30. The problem is that unless you see the individual, they will show up as obese on a local or national statistic.

'What the BVI will be able to do is look at the different sections of the body, calculate the body volumes, and give you a better idea of whether that person is truly obese.'

Clearly, that's important if you are filling in a health insurance form, applying for a job, or waiting for a hip replacement op, but how does it help the patient lose weight?

'It still depends very much on the individual,' says Dr Rahim, shaking his head as though it is an uphill struggle. 'Some people are prepared to make lifestyle changes and get their head around some of the issues that made them overweight in the first place. Whereas others have more complex relationships with food – emotional dependencies, problems, stresses, eating behaviours – routines that are just not conducive to weight loss. So you very much have to consider a person as an individual before coming up with a strategy for them, and then constantly monitor their progress and keep them enthused. Different people want to lose weight for different reasons. One size doesn't fit all.'

Dr Rahim is adamant that obesity is not anyone's 'fault'. Nor is it a sign of laziness or stupidity. Many of his patients are clever, successful people who cannot get a grip on this one problem. He reckons they need psychological help more than a diet sheet.

'I see so many people who "comfort eat" or eat for emotional reasons, many of which they don't understand themselves. You have to try and address the underlying issues. Psychological and behavioural therapies are probably more appropriate for those patients than dietary advice. The thing that you find with that cohort of people is that they already know what is good and what is bad; they're educated – they can tell you how many calories are in x, y and z – so it's not a lack of education that is stopping them losing weight; it's the other issues that are causing them problems. Unless you address those underlying issues, it's going to be difficult for that individual not only to lose weight, but to maintain that weight loss long term.

❝ Obesity is as much a social disease as a medical one – if not more so. ❞

'It partly relates to all the social changes that have occurred over the past 20 to 30 years – the abundance of processed, high-sugar, high-fat convenience food. And it also relates to our increasingly sedentary lifestyle.

'I think the way our bodies are designed is that our default position is to try and do as little physical activity and retain as many calories as possible. So to say that a whole population is lazy and greedy is not the case. It is very much a social problem for us all to tackle rather than an individual one.'

Yet so many patients beat themselves up about it. Perhaps, says Dr Rahim, doctors are to blame:

'Some patients do think they are personally to blame, they call themselves thick, lazy and stupid. "I must be," they say, "because look at me – I'm so fat!" This negativity actually impedes progress because they honestly believe they will never succeed. I believe some of that attitude comes straight from the medical professionals who treat them. They come to us for help, and all we give them is a diet sheet and the advice to eat less and exercise more, as though it is that easy. We set them up for failure, when actually the problem is almost impossible for them to solve alone.

'If you live in an area where you can't go out at night, where you've got nowhere to walk to, where there's only convenience food, which is cheap for you to buy as opposed to fresh fruit and vegetables, you're going to take the options you have and not those you might prefer.

'It is like asking them to swim against the tide, fighting against what now is classed as the social norm, with convenience foods, etc. and low levels of physical activity. That's what happens in everyday society now, and you are asking people to work against that, which most people can do for three months, maybe even six, but after that it becomes unbelievably hard.'

As a former fattie who has tried again and again, and who knows how very hard it is to lose weight, it made me feel better to hear it from a professional. It's not that fatties want an excuse. But it so helps to have a reason! A reason, a scientific explanation, of why it is so very difficult to lose weight once you have put it on. But as I travelled from city to city, and even from country to continent, to interview the world's real obesity experts, I found more and more 'reasons' and less and less 'blame'.

It quickly became apparent to me that the hardened critics in our society, who so love to blame, ridicule and patronise, have got obesity completely wrong. The media, the effortlessly slim, the worthies, even government ministers, pontificate from a position of scientific and medical ignorance.

❝ Overwhelmingly, the experts refused to talk about 'fault' – except that obesity was perhaps to be blamed upon our collective lifestyle and culture. ❞

Given that collective responsibility, which you could shorthand to 'Western lifestyle', it was simple science that was making many of us fat. And, in many cases, it was sheer luck that was keeping some of us skinny.

Magnetic resonance imaging

Now it's time to meet the Fat Team – an unprepossessing name for a group of dedicated and seriously clever clinicians (doctors who treat people, shake hands and use 'bedside manner') and scientists (those with thick-rimmed glasses and computer skills!) at London's Imperial College, who are trying to find out all about fat and how to beat it. They already know that genes play a large part:

* Many of us simply can't help having bodies that want to put on weight.
* Being fat is not your fault – but it is your problem.

That's the verdict of Professor Jimmy Bell, head of the Fat Team. Who isn't fat at all, by the way. That's despite the fact that every Tuesday is rumoured to be Cake Day in the MRI (magnetic resonance imaging) unit, deep in the bowels of Hammersmith Hospital. Here the team looks at people's fat – on the inside. And they have discovered a new breed of human being – the TOFI – who is Thin Outside, Fat Inside. Who looks slim outwardly, but who has the worst kind of fat – the visceral stuff – wrapped around, or marbled through, the inner organs. Who proves that being sanctimoniously slim may be a fraud. Because here the Fat Team have found size zero models who have dangerous amounts of fat – on the inside. And sumo wrestlers who are *not* fat on the inside – who, despite their outward obesity, are essentially healthy.

The team's work has turned the fat rationale upside down – or rather, inside out. Using the MRI scanner at Hammersmith Hospital, they can accurately pinpoint fat, precisely quantify it, and produce a staggering statistic, not in inches or pounds, but in litres.

'Our work so far has shown that you can take two men of the same age with the same BMI and find one with 5 litres of fat within him and another with 2 litres,' said Professor Bell. 'We've even scanned people who are underweight and found up to 7 litres of fat inside them! It proves how unreliable BMI is, but it also shows that, on a personal level, we need to think about our health in an entirely different way.

« You can be fat and healthy. You can be thin and unhealthy. Outward signs say nothing. What matters is your lifestyle. »

The Imperial College team has found that the average male has 5.4 litres of visceral fat, and women have 3.08 litres. But women carry more fat overall, mostly on the thighs. The total amount of fat in the average woman is 37 litres, and 30 litres for men.

'What we don't yet possess is enough information about how different genetic groups store fat. But we do know that you can manipulate the way the body stores it by changing the diet,' Professor Bell tells me.

Ah! Now we're getting somewhere. So we can change where we put fat on?

'Over the past five years we've demonised fat and become obsessed with obesity, which is mostly talked about in terms of weight loss. But what matters is where it is distributed. As you lose weight, it tends to go from the top and bottom of your body first, so it can become concentrated in the abdomen. That is the most dangerous zone of all, and it's possible that going on a constant series of diets actually encourages the storage of fat in this region.'

Suddenly the tightness of my size 16 jeans starts to make sense. I don't know about you, but over the years I have built up a wardrobe full of clothes in various sizes. I have jeans in every size from 12 to 20. I long to get back into the 12s. Every so often I stroke them adoringly.

But if yo-yo dieting actually causes you to store more fat in the abdomen, then surely the career slimmer's whole lifestyle, rotating as it does around burn and bust, binge and diet, is causing more harm than good?

'Fat cells are extremely intelligent and resistant,' says Professor Bell. 'They hang on stubbornly even through crash diets. They are the body's key survival mechanism, and they see dieting as death, so they resist at all costs. That's their job.'

Intelligent? Fat?

FAT FACTS

So what exactly is this substance that evolution gave us to keep us alive through famine and disaster, and that we have come to abhor in the modern era? How come we now hate what was once our key to survival? Professor Bell told me:

Fat cells are formed inside you in the first trimester of gestation and again during puberty. Generally, people don't generate any more in adulthood unless they more than double their weight, or if they have liposuction.

A lean adult has about 40 billion fat cells, which expand and reduce as energy is stored and used. The overweight adult can have from 75 billion to over 300 billion, depending on how obese they are.

Fat cells are all over our body and they are designed to store energy for the body to use later – even weeks later. The energy you use to run today's race may be coming from a meal you ate a month ago. Every excess calorie that your body does not use immediately as energy is stored in the fat cells – that includes calories from both healthy foods, such as fruit and vegetables, and less healthy ones, such as white bread or ice cream.

Fat cells form everywhere in the body except the brain and spinal cord. As too many of us know, they prosper in the abdomen, buttocks, breasts, thighs and upper arms. But they also encircle internal organs, cushion the eyeballs, lubricate the lungs and act like shock-absorbers on fingertips and toes.

Fat cells are rather like chemical factories, producing other substances that can cause huge long-term harm. They contribute to diabetes, heart disease, high blood pressure, strokes and other illnesses, including some cancers. As you put on more weight, the cells grow bigger. If you more than double your normal body weight, they may send out messages to nearby immature cells to divide and produce more fat cells.

Fat cells live for about 10 years – unlike brain cells, which never get replaced, or cells in the intestine, which live and die within a week. But when fat cells die they are immediately replaced, so your overall number shouldn't change.

Fat cells shrink but don't disappear. When obese people lose a great deal of weight, they don't seem to lose their total number of fat cells – the cells simply shrink and sit there, waiting to be fattened up again.

Liposuction has no effect whatsoever on health, even when surgeons suck out 20 lb or more of fat (it tackles only the subcutaneous kind). But a person who loses that much weight through dieting and exercise

will almost certainly see significant changes in blood pressure, cholesterol and insulin resistance. Liposuction also fails to shrink the fat cells
left behind.

Our shape – apple or pear – is usually genetic, but also hormonal. Men
tend to be apples, so are fatter around the middle and therefore more
at risk than those built like pears (usually women), who carry their fat
in the hips, thighs and backside. However, yo-yo dieting may change
the way the body lays down fat, and may increase the amount of toxic
visceral fat.

So what about fat intelligence?

'Well, it appears to be pretty clever stuff!' laughs Professor Bell,
who doesn't have too much of it, so he can afford to be admiring.

'For years, we thought of fat as a kind of passive storage, but
now we can see it's much more like a dynamic organ. Fat cells are
chemical factories, spewing hormones and other substances out
into the bloodstream. This has profound and sometimes harmful
effects on metabolism, weight and overall health.

'Also, it is reactive. It changes its behaviour according to what's
going on in the body. And that's where it gets exciting because we
think we can manipulate it – for example, by nutrition. It would
appear that nutritional alterations, such as eating more resistant
starch, as in lentils and pulses, means less fat is likely to be laid
down in the abdomen. We are carrying out a trial right now on
healthy volunteers to see what happens to their internal deposits of
fat when they switch to a diet involving more grains and lentils.'

And Professor Bell and his team have Superman vision when
it comes to viewing the human body. Their pictures of where and
what type of fat is stored are alarmingly clear.

Points to remember

Researchers are constantly trying to decipher the biology of fat cells, hoping to find new ways of helping people get rid of excess fat or, at least, prevent obesity from destroying their health. In an increasingly obese world, their efforts have taken on added importance. Their conclusions can be summarised as follows:

1   Only exercise gets rid of visceral fat.

2   It may help to face your demon, so look at yourself in a mirror, or try to get yourself scanned.

3   Don't dismiss fat as just a superficial problem – it could be affecting your internal organs.

4   Skinny people with unhealthy lifestyles can actually be more at risk than you, so don't accept the teasing and insults. Fat does not necessarily mean unhealthy, and skinny does not necessarily mean healthy.

5   Obesity has nothing to do with being lazy or stupid. It's a social problem, and, sadly, you are part of a bigger picture. It's not your fault. Stop blaming yourself; it will only hold you back.

6   You must change your lifestyle. At present, yours is making you fat.

7   'Comfort eaters' must look at the underlying issues. Consider seeing a psychologist/therapist, and also see page 214.

8   Those who tell you 'It's not rocket science' and 'It's easy to lose weight' are wrong. It's complex – and highly individual.

9   Stop yo-yo dieting – it could be causing you to build up extra layers of visceral fat.

10   Have yourself a bowl of lentil soup and eat more grains. We don't know yet if they help reduce visceral fat, but they can only be good for you!

BUDDYING BRINGS THE BEST RESULTS

When I first set up my weight-loss website, I called it Fat Happens. Good title, I thought, because I wanted to stress that for many people, fat does just seem to come out of nowhere. You know, like shit happens? It happens, it's horrible, it's just one of those things that life throws at you and you have to get on.

Most people liked it. A few critics pointed out that fat didn't just happen to anyone: it is caused by eating too much and exercising too little. (There are always those who love to point that out, aren't there? As if we hadn't figured it out for ourselves long ago?) But after the first year, and the first 10,000 members, I started to realise that quite another dynamic was taking over and giving the website a bright, new sense of community. That was the buddying element – a unique feature – where members can buddy up with like minds (and like bodies too) and slim together, set each other goals, keep each other on message. Even if they live miles apart and can only get together at two in the morning...

Time and again, members' emails showed how lonely they felt in their fight against fat, and how much better it was to do it with a friend. That's why I changed the name to BuddyPower. The power of a pal can be a very strong force indeed. A sympathetic and empathetic mate can keep you on track. When you think about it, making such a buddy is the first 'baby step' towards changing your own environment to one that will better support the New You.

Obesity specialists have known the value of buddying for years. The simple fact is that unless you arm yourself with buddy power, you're almost doomed to fail. The famous Dr Phil on American TV won't even accept fatties on to his weight-loss programme unless they have a small army of friends, family and even co-workers prepared to help. He likes to meet them too, and warn them of their responsibility.

Unless you have demonstrable buddy power, he won't take you on...

'I thought I was the only idiot who couldn't lose weight,' so many members blog. 'But finding a friend has made all the difference!'

I like to talk of 'buddying, not bullying' because there's no one way to lose weight and regain your health (as has been preached in the past by diet fascists). You often have to find your own tailor-made method, follow your own path, make your own journey. The era of the 'one size fits all' diet is over. Let's get fit by dancing on its grave!

WAKE UP, WHITEHALL!

＊

Before embarking on this book I went to see Iain Duncan Smith, the former leader of the Conservative party. I'd heard him speaking on the radio about 'Breakdown Britain' – how our society is suffering with families shattered by drink, drugs, bad housing and so on. As I was listening, I kept wondering, 'When is he going to mention obesity?' because it impacts upon the quality of so many lives. Yet he didn't mention it once.

This is the man who's said to be producing the report upon which David Cameron will format his future social policies. So I contacted him, and asked to meet.

He was welcoming and kind as we talked in his very swish, ruby red and shiny mahogany offices in the House of Commons. But clearly he knew nothing about fat and the misery it's causing.

'Obesity?' he asked, as he poured coffee and offered me a biscuit, which I virtuously declined. 'Is it a problem?'

Yes, I said. It could bankrupt the NHS as well as ruin the lives of the majority of families in his Broken Britain.

'Well,' he responded, 'I suppose we all put on a pound or two at Christmas, and then you never quite get rid of it again, do you?'

And that appeared to be the sum of his interest. Honestly – I'm not being selective or biased, and I am hardly editing the encounter at all. There was lots of courtesy, but I detected no interest. Perhaps he hadn't read any of the headlines, or seen the ordinary men and women outside in Westminster Square. Perhaps no one in his family was fed up with a fat problem that they couldn't shift.

Cripes, I thought. If they get in at the next election, Britain will be the fattest nation on Earth within months, and the NHS, which the Tories claim to hold dear, will explode through over-consumption and die.

I went away, feeling rather depressed, and wrote him an email – which was never even acknowledged. But I had to try, in my own layperson's terms, to outline to him why obesity is *not* just a health matter, and why it is very much part of his Broken Britain.

Dear Mr Duncan Smith

The obesity epidemic isn't just a health issue – it impacts upon a number of different government departments.

First and foremost – Health: People don't die of obesity per se, but they do die of its 'co-morbidities', including heart disease, cancer, stroke, etc. Quality of life is diminished through immobility and related disease. It has been likened by some to alcoholism, and requires similarly holistic treatment programmes (All Party Select Committee report on Obesity, 27 May 2004). The cost of obesity was conservatively estimated by the National Audit Office (2001) to be around £3.3–£3.7 billion a year, and including overweight, around £6.6–£7.4 billion.

Education: One in five children in the UK is obese. Childhood obesity from 2004 figures published in 2006 (*Health of the*

Nation) run at approximately 19 per cent, with 25 per cent of young people between the ages of 11 and 16 being obese. We need to re-educate children in home economics, food science, cooking, PE and human biology to reverse the trend. The 2006 NICE report on obesity proposes 'policies relating to building layout and recreational spaces, catering (including vending machines) and the food and drink children bring into school, the taught curriculum (including PE), school travel plans and provision for cycling'.

Work & Pensions: Obesity reduces productivity, cuts short working life and increases demand for incapacity benefits.

Transport: Prevention of obesity must be considered in future plans, i.e. sustainable cycle paths, types of public transport, etc.

Environment: Britain's streets and cities must become consumer-friendly and more conducive to walking, cycling and fitness pursuits, providing facilities and schemes such as cycling and walking routes, cycle parking, area maps and safe play areas. The 2006 NICE report proposes 'making streets cleaner and safer through measures such as traffic calming, congestion charging, pedestrian crossings, cycle routes, lighting and walking schemes; ensuring buildings and spaces are designed to encourage people to be more physically active (for example, through positioning and signposting of stairs, entrances and walkways).

DEFRA: Britain actually suffers from malnutrition. Food is plentiful, but is mostly processed, high in fats, sugar and salt, and low in fibre, calcium, vitamins and iron. Such a diet is conducive to weight gain and ill health. The junk food industry can be compared to the tobacco industry 50 years ago – reluctant to make changes unless forced to do so, and advertising and selling a product that can be damaging to health. The diet industry should be similarly considered.

The Treasury: Lost tax revenue from loss of employment, reduced life expectancy of the workforce, and additional costs to the NHS.

Obesity directly impacts on many of the main concerns highlighted in 'Breakdown Britain', including poverty, depression, poor quality of life, changed family dynamics, ill health and prejudice. The approach, therefore, must be two-pronged: prevention *plus* the treatment of a generation already suffering.

Obesity is having a disastrous effect upon the health of the nation, and government is slow to tackle it, addressing in the simplest terms prevention of obesity for a new generation of children, whilst 'writing off' a whole generation of adults and teenagers who are too expensive and difficult to help. In my opinion, government is consumed by a paralysis of fear over this issue. However, according to NICE:

'*If current trends of overweight and obesity continue, the Department of Health (Zaninotto et al., 2006) have estimated that by 2010, the number of people overweight and obese in England could increase by 14%. Therefore it could be assumed the costs could rise to between £7.5 and £8.4 billion per year.*

'*Therefore it could be assumed that reducing obesity by 1% or preventing a 1% increase in obesity would result in cost avoidance of between £66 and £74 million per year.*'

At present, 20 million voters are obese – and the vast majority are desperately seeking a way out of their plight.

Yours sincerely
Anne Diamond

CHAPTER 3

IS THERE REALLY AN OBESITY EPIDEMIC?

✳

W ell, I had to ask the question, didn't I? Even though it seems to be universally accepted that fat is happening almost everywhere around the world, and that the media, the NHS and even government now talk about the obesity epidemic as fact. Even though I am now patron of the National Obesity Forum here in the UK, whose foundation is more or less based on the shocking statistic that one in four women and one in five men in Britain is obese. Even though it's reckoned that a quarter of our children are at risk of getting too fat for their health, and destined to become unfit, unhappy and unhealthy adults.

I started by asking one of the world's loudest voices in the field of weight, who claims exactly the opposite – that an obesity epidemic is largely a myth, and that a smaller, social problem is being grossly inflated by medics, politicians and the diet industry who want to control our lives, frighten us into submission and further exploit us. It sounds to me as if he's saying that the obesity epidemic is a conspiracy of grotesque proportions, and we simply play into the hands of the plotters by discussing it at all.

He's Patrick Basham, and you can think what you like about his views, but his pedigree is as impressive as his writings are volatile, challenging and extreme! He's an expat Brit, a Channel

Islander, who lectures on health policy at America's Johns Hopkins University and founded the Democracy Institute, a politically independent London- and Washington-based public policy research organisation. He founded the Social Affairs Centre at the Fraser Institute, Canada's leading think tank, and he's written books and hundreds of magazine and newspaper articles about health, diet and obesity. His latest book, *Diet Nation: Exposing the Obesity Crusade*, came out in December 2006, and questioned just about everything currently being said about obesity and how it's affecting our health.

He's seriously worried about the nanny state – about chilling armies of Gestapo-like inspectors tearing the lids off our children's lunch-boxes to scrutinise what Mum has put inside. He fears for our liberty to be whatever weight we want without the scorn of a judgemental and even punitive society. He dreads a world dominated by the 'thin is everything' culture, and warns against us all becoming its victims. And there he has a point, doesn't he? Civil liberties, even those that allow us to kill ourselves slowly in the manner of our choice, are something to be defended at all costs, aren't they?

Several months ago, while I was making one of my regular appearances on TV's *The Wright Stuff*, we were discussing a hard-hitting and, in my view, indefensible, initiative by Ealing Council in London to help smokers give up their unhealthy habit. At a cost to the taxpayer of £75,000, they had formed a squad of 'Smoking Police' to stop smokers as they walked down the street minding their own business, or smoking outside betting shops, supermarkets or even at bus stops, and ask them to blow into a carbon monoxide monitor, then sign up for a stop smoking programme. In some cases, they might even be offered counselling.

'No one will be forced to do anything,' the council protested when the UK media reacted with horror. 'We reckon it could help about 2400 people to give up.'

I was immediately outraged, even though I hate smoking and the often anti-social behaviour of many smokers. This was taking the campaign too far. It is already illegal for smokers to indulge their habit in public places, but to pursue them down the street with well-meaning health tests and patronising advice? This, I suggested, was sheer harassment.

I thought how offended and hurt I would be if those health workers approached me as I was perusing the deli counter in Tesco's and interrupted my reverie: 'Excuse me, madam, but we noticed that you are a little fat – would you like to stand on these scales and appreciate the true nature of your obesity? And then perhaps you would like some leaflets on how to lose weight, or a session with a council therapist who could tell you why you have ended up in such a predicament?' Never mind offended or hurt – I would just punch them in the nose!

Not so a great many of the viewers who rang in – mostly smokers who said they were so desperate to give up, and who found it so very hard, that they actually welcomed anything else that might provide an extra stimulus. 'Maybe I need another kick up the bum,' as one put it.

So perhaps obesity too needs proactive stimulus tantamount to harassment and persecution?

'This is where Big Brother State wants to become Big Nanny State,' says Patrick Basham. He reckons politicians and the diet industry are seeking control through fear – telling us that we're all going to die unless we do things their way. And the language of control, he says, is epic in proportion. Bring on the high-definition, wide-screen, panoramic vista and the John Williams soundtrack.

'Obesity is the terror within. Unless we do something about it, the magnitude of the problem will dwarf 9/11 or any other terrorist attempt.'
US Surgeon General, 2006

'If we don't act dramatically now, our children will have shorter life spans than us for the first time in recorded history.'
Former President Bill Clinton, 2007

'Obesity will hit us harder and faster than global warming.'
Alan Johnson, UK health minister, 2007

'We are experiencing an unprecedented epidemic of life-threatening obesity.'
Professor Philip James of the International Obesity Task Force, 2005

And in 2006 the government's long-awaited 'Foresight' report predicted that half the population of the UK will be clinically obese within 25 years, and that by 2050 obesity will cost the country £45 billion a year. Enough to wreck the National Health Service. There's no doubt, if you believe the forecasts, the outlook does indeed look dismal.

Patrick Basham shakes his head: 'The media has picked up on the scares and turned them into a kind of orthodoxy. Now everyone accepts it because they have read it so often, it must be true! For instance, the term "childhood obesity" occurred only twice in the *Guardian* in 1999. In 2004 it occurred 201 times, almost four times a week. The public have become convinced that the "epidemic" is a fact.'

Basham reckons that claims of an epidemic in the UK, or even the USA, are 'wildly exaggerated' to suit the agenda of empire-building politicians, public-health bureaucrats and big business, including the pharmaceutical industry.

'They preach a sermon consisting of four obesity myths: that we and our children are fat; that being fat is a certain recipe for early death; that our fatness stems from the manufacturing and marketing practices of the food industry; and that we will lengthen our lives if only we eat less and lose weight. The trouble is, there is no scientific evidence to support these claims.

'The people that I then worry about are those who listen to it all, become disillusioned and unhappy with their bodies, and condemn themselves to lives of yo-yo dieting and an unhealthy obsession with getting thin at all costs.'

Basham reminds me that a poll of 5000 British women for *Grazia* magazine in 2006 found that four in 10 had suffered from an eating disorder, such as anorexia or bulimia.

'While we are being fed the notion that our fatness is going to kill us unless we demonise the food industry, ban certain foods, ban the advertising of more, and all go on a diet, the truth about the risks of thinness and the large number of thinness-related deaths is quietly ignored. Large numbers of women suffer from anorexia, with one in five hospital cases ending in death.'

I start to see where he is coming from. He tells me his next book is called *Dying to Diet: A Practitioner's Personal Story*.

'It analyses the dieting culture that underpins – and the diet industry that largely underwrites – the anti-obesity campaign,' he adds. 'I am writing the book in concert with my sister. She is a London-based osteopath and, most tellingly, a lifelong sufferer from eating disorders. For her, the writing is proving to be a cathartic exercise. We trust that our book will help the "thin is everything" culture's large number of female (and, increasingly, male) victims.'

The erosion of personal choice, the demonising of fat, the investment in possibly erroneous, misguided and ineffective campaigns, the peril of worshipping thinness – I understand those dangers. They are very real. But so is the simple truth facing every schoolteacher I know.

In the classroom

Ten, perhaps 15 years ago, there was possibly one fat child per class. You knew it because he was often the one singled out by the bullies. Nowadays, there are many fat children in class. It's almost the norm – it's certainly not unusual. Even in the relatively affluent area of Oxford where I live, one head teacher told me she was worried, and depressed, about the level of obesity in her primary school, and was deliberately taking action to provide more playtime.

'They don't run around like they used to,' she told me. 'But what can I do? Our playing fields were sold off years ago, and we just have a small tarmac area for a bit of skipping and pavement games. It's not like when I was at school – we had a field that was so long we used to run out of teachers' earshot. And that was still in an inner city.

'If your expert doesn't think there is an epidemic, he should come here and use his eyes. But I understand his concern about anorexia, too. A great many of our little girls talk about nothing else than how to be as thin as the celebrities they see on TV. We caught some of them encouraging others to go to the chemist with them after school to try and buy slimming pills.'

Patrick Basham's answer is to concentrate, not upon food and its possible over-consumption, but upon exercise and why we live more sedentary lives than we ever used to. One expert I spoke to in Birmingham, Dr David Ashton, agrees.

'Demonising the food industry is not the answer,' he said. 'We need to get people out more. If I could convince all my patients to spend every lunchtime going for an hour's walk, then we wouldn't have anything like the scale of the problem we see today.'

Instead, according to Basham, for the first time in many years British gyms are not as popular as they used to be. Yet another survey showed that women prefer to diet, choose slimming pills, starve themselves or even consider surgery than take up exercise. Are we becoming lazy, or simply more accustomed to a sedentary lifestyle? Perhaps we have become disillusioned with the gymnasium fad – after all, it is *so* boring and repetitive! And expensive. Yes, that might have something to do with it too.

Yet there's one sad fact put forward by the anti-obesity crusade that even Basham does not deny. Most attempts to lose weight (at least through dieting) end in failure, even in highly controlled situations. Of every 100 people who give it a go, only four will be able to maintain their post-diet weight. Ninety-five per cent of dieters are fatter five years after their diet then when they started to slim. That explains a lot to me! Does it ring true to you too?

All of this should be music to the ears of any self-assured, totally content, proud-to-be-fattie. But the truth is, I haven't met many of them. Actually I have never, ever met one fat man, woman or child who wanted to be anything other than slim. I've met quite a few who make the best of being overweight – who keep themselves fit, and have a positive, happy attitude to life. But they'd all rather be slim. If I could invent a pill that would, without fail, turn a fattie into a slimmie overnight, I guarantee everyone would want to take it.

Is Patrick, then – and others like him, who say the 'epidemic' is a myth designed to make yet more money out of us and 'hook' us into a dieting culture – guilty of burying his head in the sand?

After all, hasn't he been to Disneyworld? Hasn't he seen the mountains of flab in skimpy shorts and marvelled at the hour-long queues of obese holidaymakers (surely they cannot all be disabled) at the scooter rental? Pay $40 for a day's electric mobility, and you get to skip to the front of the line at each ride. If there is any one place in the world you could truly witness the consequences of the super-size culture, surely Florida's playground is the best vantage point...

'Yes, I've seen them,' says Patrick, 'and I don't deny obesity is a bigger problem than it once was. But an epidemic? It is true that body mass index statistics show a significant increase in overweight adults over the past decade. But they moved the goalposts! In 1997 the BMI classification of being overweight was changed from 27 to 25. At a stroke, millions of people previously classed as normal suddenly became overweight, with no good reason to explain the change. In fact, the average adult weighs only a pound or two more than 20-odd years ago. Yes, there's an increase in the morbidly obese – those with a BMI greater than 40 – but they make up less than 5 per cent. What's more, there are even statistics which show that we are actually eating fewer calories on average than we used to 30 years ago.'

Dr Colin Waine, of the National Obesity Forum, vehemently disagrees:

'You can skew statistics how you please, but there is no doubt that British men, women and children are getting bigger – that obesity kills, and ruins the quality of life. We have a very unhealthy relationship with food, and the food industry should be held to account for promoting unhealthy eating, particularly in our children.

'Inaction on this issue will kill us. That's the truth, plain and simple. You must make whatever choice, personally, that you wish. But as a society, we have to care enough to do something to make it easier for people to get healthy.'

FAT IS NOW THE NORM...

Do you really have to hit rock bottom before you'll get the impetus to change? I was interviewing a weight-loss hypnotist recently, who reckons that the only way some fatties will ever find the motivation to make real and lasting changes to their lifestyle is if he can get them to revisit the most painful experience caused by their obesity.

Isn't it painful enough for them already, just being fat, I protested? Doesn't the world beat us up enough?

'No,' he said. 'The trouble is, it's becoming the norm to be fat. And the media is so keen to show us images of unusually obese people – you know, the sort that have to be airlifted out of their own homes to go to hospital, or the infants who weigh more than their parents – that the "ordinary obese" reassure themselves that they're not too bad.'

It's a worrying vision. With the prediction that by 2015 just over half the UK population could be dangerously fat, perhaps we're on a hopeless downward spiral. The more of us who get fat, the more acceptable it will become, so the fatter we'll get...

My friend the hypnotist therefore takes his patients back to that dreadful moment when fat turned to pain, or embarrassment, or downright humiliation. And he makes them wallow in it. Like getting wedged into your airline seat and needing help to disembark. Or having a restaurant chair collapse under you. Or breaking the cross-trainer at the gym. Or being refused a camel ride on holiday in Egypt because you might break the camel's back! All these things actually happened to members of BuddyPower.com, my weight-loss support website. But one recent posting showed the real, everyday pain of being fat. It was from a young woman who described her oh-so-perfect life:

'I'm Lizzie, I'm 41, slim, attractive and in control of things. I enjoy inline skating, horse-riding and mucking about on the trampoline with my three gorgeous kids. I live in the countryside and walk the dogs in my novelty wellies. In summer I often pop round to the neighbours to use their pool and love getting together with the girls in their hot tubs for a glass of wine and a gossip. I enjoy clubbing in Ibiza with my gay friends in the summer, and have lots of wonderful friends and a lovely husband who adores me. In short, I love my life.'

Sounds a pretty good life, doesn't it? Lizzie had me going green with envy. Sadly, she then went on to admit that it was only partially true, the rest a distant dream. Yes, she had the lovely kids, husband and friends. But being obese tainted her enjoyment of nearly everything else. Her knees hurt too much to skate. She can't get wellies around her 'enormous' calves. She dreads being asked to the pool parties, and lives in permanent fear of the disparaging remarks made by the neighbours' kids. 'As outwardly confident as I am,' she bemoaned, 'I struggle answering, "Why do your legs look funny?" and "Do you have a baby in your tummy?" or having to hear, "Mummy, why is Lizzie so fat?" from behind a towel.'

Lizzie is resolute, though. She says she's been on a long, rough journey with her weight, but this time she is going to reach the finish. My heart goes with her. I don't know whether wallowing in the pain of these experiences would help much, though.

We must all find our own motivation because fat is no way to live. Never mind the global statistics: is beating our own personal obesity crisis going to be a challenge only self-help can cure?

Burying the problem

Nowhere is the tragedy of the global problem more plainly displayed than in a tiny, 'one-horse' town in Randolph County, Indiana, USA. It's called Lynn, and it's a great little town to raise kids 'as long as you're willing to drive at least 10 minutes to get to anything bigger than the small-town grocery store'. Lynn has no red-amber-green traffic lights and no fast food; it has one grocery store, one Co-Op, one car wash, two banks, two petrol stations, and at least six churches. Its claim to fame is a local, family-owned company called Goliath Casket.

Goliath, started in 1985 by Pee Wee Davis, who was the first to recognise a new trend, is a business that specialises in making oversize coffins. He'd noticed an upsurge in demand for coffins for the obese, and he was only too aware that their needs were not being met. So he left his job as a welder in another coffin factory and said, 'Boys, I'm gonna go home and build oversize caskets that you would be proud to put your mother in.'

Goliath started producing double-wide caskets for sale all over the USA, but has now found a growing need for 'triple-width' models. Fifteen years ago they averaged one triple-wide a year: now it's five per month.

A standard coffin is 2 feet wide, whereas the triple-width is a staggering 3 feet 8 inches. So, as you can imagine, hearses have had to be redesigned. Bigger cemetery plots have to be booked. The monster coffin business is booming. Recently, they had to build one that was 6 feet 7 inches wide – for a 64-stone man who died in Alaska. It's bigger than a king-size bed, and steel reinforced.

Pee Wee's son, Keith, runs the company now, with his wife, Juliane. Keith has written a series of articles for funeral homes on the logistics of obese funerals. He is compassionate towards the obese because he's only too aware of the problems obesity causes:

'One woman ended up face-down in her casket after the body lift broke. Another funeral home could not get the casket through the door. Then there was the casket that creaked and buckled during the service as it teetered on a small stand. And there was the casket that couldn't close, which ended up on the evening news. That family called us in tears. Some families are forced to buy two graves. Others have to use pick-up trucks to transport a coffin to the cemetery. One service was held in a garage.

'I have to stop myself walking up to people in restaurants and telling them to put away their second helpings. There's no reason for anyone in this country not to have a good diet. If everyone went on a diet, I could find something else to do!'

It's happening here in the UK too. Bigger crematorium furnaces are now being built all over Britain, and undertakers are having to build bigger coffins. Even five years ago, it was rare to have a coffin that couldn't be physically carried. Now that happens every single week – that's according to John Weir of the UK Funeral Directors Union. The combined weight of a casket and large corpse now regularly exceeds 47 stone.

Who's the fattest?

Statistics are constantly changing, and no country really wants to admit that its population is leading the field in terms of obese citizens. However, the figures show some alarming trends in perhaps surprising places, so it's as well to take note. But statistics can also be confusing. The USA, for example, has a lower percentage of obese folk than a tiny Pacific Island, but because it is such a huge country, the number of actual sufferers is immense.

Australia

Given its healthy, outdoor image, it comes as a shock to learn that Australia recently became the fattest nation on Earth, with more obese citizens than any other single country. However, many of my Australian experts vehemently deny this, saying there's no way they could be fatter than the USA. But the latest figures do conclude that around 4 million Australian adults, or 26 per cent of the adult population, are obese, prompting Professor Simon Stewart, author of *Australia's Future 'Fat Bomb'*, to complain: 'We could fill the Melbourne Cricket Ground 40 times over with the number of obese Australians now, and you can double that if you look at the people who are also overweight. If we ran a Fat Olympics, we'd be gold medal winners as the fattest people on Earth at the moment.'

If the crisis is not averted, Aussie obesity experts have warned, health costs could top $6 billion, and an extra 700,000 people will be admitted to hospital for heart attacks, strokes and blood clots caused by excess weight.

Boyd Swinburn, Australia's leading child obesity expert, told me he blames the sort of inaction feared by Colin Waine of the UK National Obesity Forum. 'The previous federal government blamed parents and individuals and told them to pull up their socks. All that's done is make us fatter as a nation,' he said.

France

Who'd have thought it? The French, famous for their healthy Mediterranean diet, are getting fat, though nowhere near the scale of Americans, Britons or Australians. An estimated 55,000 people in France die of obesity-related illnesses every year. In 2005 even the winner of *Star Academy*, their *Pop Idol* equivalent, was a sensation, not because of her voice, but because of her size. Aged 19, pretty Magalie Bonneau was 5 feet 1 inch tall and 11½ stone. She was dubbed the 'heavyweight' of French TV channel TF1, and put under enormous pressure to slim. Sound familiar? She eventually lost 29 lb under the pressure of her new-found fame, but she has been keen to point out that 'French audiences are getting used to seeing plump girls'.

More recently, the French have come up with a stark poster, designed to terrify the fat off you. It shows a picture of abject depression, a hugely obese and naked woman, hunched over in despair. Above her are printed the words: '*L'obésité tue. Ça vous fait toujours marrer?*' (Obesity kills. Still think it's a laughing matter?)

FRENCH WOMEN DON'T GET FAT?

I was on a TV show recently, debating whether or not there really is an obesity epidemic. It's rapidly getting like sparring with that bunch of conspiracy theorists who claim that Apollo 11 never really landed on the moon, and it was all a giant hoax played out by NASA to gain cold war prestige.

There are a few so-called eminent scientists and doctors who reckon obesity is an extremist and alarming hype, actively encouraged by the diet and drugs industry and doctors in their pay, who will happily profit from a scare. They're right to be sceptical, of course. There have been many eras in history when fat has been both desirable and celebrated, and the global population has not suffered any ill effects. But surely what is happening nowadays is entirely different?

I was still pondering this as I received a ton of letters following the TV programme. One very kind lady sent me a well-thumbed book to which she'd attached a note: 'Read this, Anne, and you'll see that there's no excuse for being fat. All it needs is a different attitude.' The book was the famous, and now infamous, *French Women Don't Get Fat!* – the best-seller that claimed to explain the 'French paradox' of beautiful, chic French women eating massive three-course meals every day and yet staying slim and gorgeous. It supposedly teaches you the 'life of indulgence without bulge, satisfying yen without yo-yo on three meals a day'. Yes, the book is witty and often wise, but its title is hopelessly out of date because French women *are* getting fat, I have learnt. And yes, I was shocked too! Official statistics now state that 11.3 per cent of the French are obese, with nearly another 40 per cent overweight. OK, that's puny compared to the obesity stats from the USA, or even the UK. But the French! *Zut alors!*

They used to be known for market freshness and old-fashioned cooking with flair. Things are changing, however. Now they have British- and American-style supermarkets and convenience foods, and they're using microwaves (*sacré bleu!*) in schools, offices and homes. Their own government reckons that the average French mealtime, which used to average one hour and 20 minutes, now takes just 38 minutes. McDonald's and Kentucky Fried Chicken are planning to open dozens of new stores throughout France this year. WeightWatchers, which only started France in 1992, now sells 3000 tons of frozen food every year to would-be French slimmers.

The changing shape in France is a bit of a blow to the nature/nurture theorists too. Apparently, many scientists reckoned French people didn't get fat because they had no fat gene. In a country that has always enjoyed abundance, perhaps French *Homo sapiens* never needed to develop one. Sadly, the 21st century is disproving that idea.

Now the French government is targeting *le snack*, and all advertisements for products considered unhealthy are accompanied by health warnings about the dangers of eating too much fat, salt and sugar. It's a sure sign that no country can afford to be complacent.

India

In India, alongside the problems of starvation and malnutrition, there is a new malaise – and it seems obscene by comparison. Obesity now affects some 5 per cent of the population and yes, they are calling it an epidemic, particularly among the wealthier middle classes. For the first time in human history the number of overweight people in India, 2.1 billion, is equal to the number of underweight people, says Dr Pradeep Chowbey, an Indian surgeon who has a queue of wealthy middle-class men and women outside his surgery, waiting for gastric bands and bypasses.

Dr Anoop Mishra, head of the Indian Obesity Task Force, put it bluntly: 'Nowadays Indian kids spend more time watching cricket on TV than playing it outside. Something fundamental has changed within our society.' They even have a slimming competition, *India's Biggest Loser*, on TV, drawing record audiences and millions of applications from contestants hoping to win 100,000 rupees (£1700).

Oxfam report an emerging concern they call 'nutrition transition', where a developing country can go from starvation to obesity without ever going through a period of normality. They say it is not a disease of affluence; it is a disease of globalisation, and talk about the spread of the 'Westernised' lifestyle.

It does make you wonder. Not to point the finger in any way whatsoever at McDonald's, who will not hesitate to litigate if they feel unfairly treated, and suffer a great deal of criticism when it comes to the obesity/fast food debate, there is a story worth telling that speaks volumes about the 'Westernised lifestyle', and I'll leave you to wonder about the burgers...

Japan

In 1971 in Tokyo, when they opened the first McDonald's in Japan, the new director of the company, Den Fujita, reportedly told journalists: 'The reason Japanese people are so short and have yellow skins is because they have eaten nothing but fish and rice for two thousand years. If we eat McDonald's hamburgers and potatoes for a thousand years, we will become taller, our skin become white and our hair blonde.' (Love 1995) Now, in 2008, Japan has 13 million obese citizens.

China

Chinese people are becoming overweight at an alarming rate. New figures from the Health Ministry show that urban Chinese boys aged six are 2.5 inches taller and 6.6 lb heavier on average than Chinese city boys 30 years ago.

China 'has entered the era of obesity' says Ji Chengye, a leading child health researcher. 'The speed of growth is shocking.'

Today there are 20 million cars on the roads in China; six years ago there were only 6 million. Not so long ago, our familiar image of Chinese cities was of hordes of cyclists in the streets of Beijing. Now there are bumper-to-bumper cars.

Nowhere is untouched

Continue the trip around the world and the statistics become more fascinating as you go...

Croatia has the largest proportion of obese men in Europe, 31 per cent.
Albania has the most obese women, 36 per cent.
Lebanon has the largest proportion of obese men in the eastern Mediteranean, at 36 per cent.

Jordan has the eastern Mediterranean's highest female incidence of obesity, at 60 per cent.

Iran has a population of which more than half is overweight or obese. Dr Nizal Sarrafzadegan says: 'We think this is the problem of a Western lifestyle. It was not popular for people to prefer junk food, fast food, 20 years ago. Now we have a high prevalence of hypertension, diabetes, smoking and high cholesterol. Iranian children now watch an average of four hours of television a day, and adults drive cars more and exercise less than they used to.' (Saberi, 2005)

Now, as part of the doctor's Isfahan Healthy Heart Programme, mosques offer health education and exercise classes. The city bans private cars on some streets on certain days in order to encourage exercise. Pre-marriage classes now, in addition to teaching about birth control and sexually transmitted diseases, teach young men and women how to cook low-fat meals and stay fit.

FATTEST NATIONS IN THE WORLD

The most obese nations of the world per head of population are all in the western Pacific:

> **Nauru:** 80 per cent of men; 78 per cent of women
> **Tonga:** 47 per cent of men; 70 per cent of women
> **Samoa:** 33 per cent of men; 63 per cent of women

The inhabitants of these places always had a tendency to fat, but now it's getting out of control.

Military concerns

The global obesity epidemic has even hit the military, and is a source of great concern to both commanders and government.

✳ The average US soldier today is more than 22 lb heavier than his Second World War counterpart.

✳ Germany's soldiers are fatter than the average citizen: 40 per cent are overweight, compared with 35 per cent of civilians of the same age.

✳ The British army plans to extend the training period for young recruits because so many are obese. Only a third of all 16-year-olds would pass the BMI set for all recruits to the forces.

The price of obesity

Obesity costs not just lives, but money. And health economists reckon it's the commercialisation, the 'branding' of food, that's the principal cause.

'Westernised' applies not just to a type of food, but the very way foods are marketed and consumed. Many countries are now re-examining their policies concerning the advertising of food, and in particular fast food, to children. In Quebec, Canada, there are possibly the strictest rules of anywhere in the world. Basically, they've banned all direct television advertising to children – of anything, including toys. Now new studies have revealed that children in Quebec are becoming obese – but it's more prevalent among the English-speaking famillies, not the French speakers. Is this because it's only the English-speaking kids who are being influenced by US ads, which are broadcast over the border, whereas the French speakers are not even tuning in? Researchers are trying to find out.

In Australia, the issue of TV advertising and childhood obesity has been a constant battleground, with successive governments and TV companies demanding proof that a ban would work. Australian professor of children's health Boyd Swinburn, told me: 'If anyone is still unconvinced that marketing junk food works to increase kids' consumption of junk food, they just need to consider the many billions of dollars being invested annually by food companies to target kids. They do not throw away billions of dollars without the evidence that it works. Marketing works – we even teach it at universities.'

GETTING FAT IS CHILD'S PLAY

When Dreamworks made *Shrek the Third*, they created not just a storybook ogre and king, but also a great range of opportunities for commercial endorsements and product licensing, often for children's food, and it is worth a king's ransom. Before anyone even sees the movie, their offspring will already have been bombarded by Shrek sweets, cereals, biscuits and even chews that turn the mouth green.

His face, it seems, is on everything that is marketed to kids. 'His smile is synonymous with the rampant marketing of junk values,' according to one lobby group in America, who've found 17 different Shrek food promotions featuring more than 70 different products, many of which are for energy-dense, low-nutrient foods.

Yet, in the most dumbfounding of double standards, the US government's Health and Human Services Department is paying a small fortune to use Shrek to lead an anti-obesity campaign and encourage children to 'get up and play an hour a day'. Fat lot of good that'll do. Even if a generation of obese children can be prised away from the TV, they'll simply see Shrek and his erstwhile wisecracking donkey sidekick being used to sell them everything from M&Ms to PopTarts.

Did you know that the US government even allows poster advertising in school corridors and playgrounds? I know only because the state of Massachusetts has become the first to ban it!

'Surely this is a conflict of interest?' says Susan Linn, who has founded the Boston-based Campaign for a Commercial-Free Childhood. 'Can't the government find a better spokesperson for healthy living than a character that is a walking advertisement for McDonald's, sugary cereals, cookies, and candy?'

Perhaps this is what is wrong with our whole attitude towards obesity and how to beat it. We as a society don't want to face up to the truth – that our values may be wrong and we need to mend our ways. Now, as a token, we are allowing the food industry itself to spearhead campaigns for healthier living! To me it all seems pretence and simply plays into their hands, allowing them to safeguard their commercial future.

Somewhere along the line we allowed our food – the very staff of life – to become a marketable commodity, a branded commercial product. It didn't seem so bad when it was about a particular recipe for chutney or pickle ('Can anyone really make it like Branston?', launched in 1922 and still firmly embedded in the British consciousness?), or the essence of an old-fashioned English summer afternoon bottled inside Robinson's Barley Water. But now it's becoming more and more difficult to find food that doesn't have a branded label. Try buying the raw ingredients for a tuna salad and you'll soon see that it's easier to buy a ready-made version, concocted by some expert in a white coat and assembled on a production line either at downtown Tesco, Sainsbury's or M&S. There's nothing inherently wrong with any of those choices, except what they might lead to – or already have. The commercial ownership of everything – even the air we breathe. Already our water is branded. Mark my word, one day it will stop coming through the taps and then the food industry will finally have us licked.

On the news recently, what did I hear? Organic allotments in Hampshire are to be bulldozed to make way for 470 Barratt houses. Forests of scaffolding are replacing mature trees. There goes the neighbourhood! Yet as the allotments disappear, surely this of all times should be when we get out garden forks and trowels and start digging again – as our parents did in the Second World War – and dig for England's waistlines? Sorry if you've turned your back garden into a Titchmarsh paradise with a Tommy Walsh deck and a Charlie Dimmock water feature; now is the time to pull it all up and plant onions, runner beans and sweet potatoes. We need to get back to basics, and we need a multi-million pound government campaign to entreat us to take action. What's more – wouldn't it be fun? How many of our children know the unique taste and smell of a garden-grown strawberry or tomato? Tear open a bag of supermarket lettuce and all you get is a whiff of the gases injected by the packing companies to keep the produce shelf-fresh.

If we're going to tackle the obesity epidemic, we need joined-up thinking from government departments so that the approach can be two-pronged:

1   Make our environment more conducive to healthy living.
2   Take individual and personal responsibility to change what we eat and keep fit.

We must find ways forward. Perhaps we should remind the guys in charge of legislation and policy that the obesity scourge needs to be led from the front – and not left to the likes of Shrek and his cronies.

But taxing junk food won't help. Any move to do so simply shows an ignorance of the underlying causes of obesity. Health economists, such Carol Propper from Bristol University, explained to me: 'It costs the NHS £1 billion a year and the economy £2 billion through sickness and early death, rising to £45 billion by 2050. But don't tax junk food – it would just hit the poor harder. They are the biggest consumers of convenience foods. It's technology that's fattening.'

Technology – that's another part of Westernisation that seems to be proving lethal to us humans. Since the arrival of the micro-wave oven, we seem to have gone downhill. With the rise of the computer-based office job, things have gone from bad to worse. Countries we still refer to as 'third world' are nevertheless increasingly industrialised, and even in India and China, adults' and children's lifestyles have become more sedentary.

As the US-based Worldwatch Institute announced last year: 'For the first time, the number of overweight individuals worldwide rivals those who are underweight. And sadly, developing nations have joined the ranks of countries encumbered by obesity.'

It's a conundrum that seems almost obscene. As one United Nations expert told me, 'Unfortunately, food doesn't always get to the people who need it most. Hunger is one result. Obesity is another.'

WHY THE NAKED APE HAS BECOME OBESE

Desmond Morris, the zoologist turned manwatcher who catapult-
ed to world fame when he wrote *The Naked Ape* back in the 1960s,
lives just down the road from me. I have jogged breathlessly past
his house on many a frosty morning, usually at the start of yet another New Year's resolution to get fit. It has never lasted long...

I wonder if he saw me? Because he watches joggers with the
sort of reflective curiosity that spawns his many books, such as
The Human Zoo and *Peoplewatching*. He analyses the faces of
those puffing and panting past the windows of his den, and thinks:
'Are they happy joggers, or are they punishing themselves? Are
they anxious, or relaxed?' Because it matters, you see. Attitude to
life is all important, in his view.

Desmond Morris already knows that the Naked Ape is becoming more and more overweight or obese. He has seen it. But, he
holds, that doesn't mean we as a society are swirling down the toi-
let bowl of life. To lump everyone together just because of their size
would, he reckons, be unwise. And then to imagine us all doomed
would be a fallacy. Not everyone is fat for the same reason – and
it's the reasons that count. More than the fat.

This time I approach his house in a car rather than my jogging
pants. I haven't seen Desmond since he sat on my breakfast TV

sofa, back in the 1980s and '90s. Do you know, he hasn't changed a bit? I remember him in the 1950s and '60s as the presenter of *Zoo Time*, one of the first serious zoologists (he was curator of mammals at London Zoo) ever to 'go pop' and demystify an increasingly fascinating area of science for a new generation. And that's what he's been doing ever since – and still is. He's currently writing two more books to add to the 76 already in his bibliography.

'And whenever I'm writing, I put on about a stone!' he mischievously confided in me as we sat down to talk obesity and why it's happening to 21st-century man. He pats his stomach – not that it's especially noticeable.

'I'm fat at the moment because every time I write a book – and I've written three in the past two years – I put on weight. I know this is going to happen. You can't help it. When you write, you're sitting down in front of a screen or reading all the time.'

I nod in wholehearted agreement. Just writing *this* book has kept me for hours at a desk when I should have been up and about, keeping to my New Year's resolution to jog further downtown than Desmond Morris's house! I've been putting on weight because I've been writing a book about obesity. The irony is enough to boil the mercury in my blood pressure monitor.

Desmond, ever the manwatcher, has caught glimpses of himself in the mirror – and he even has a theory about the changing shape of the Naked Ape he sees reflected there.

'I like to make a curious distinction between being fat and being obese. I think a man is obese when he gets fat sideways. He's fat when he gets obese forwards. I have a big pot-belly now, but I haven't spread out on all sides. I'm still the same width, but front to back is a different story. I still take a good photograph from the front! In profile I don't want to see my image at all!'

We both laugh, and he explains:

'My defence, your honour, is that Churchill had a pot-belly, was quite podgy and lived to 90. And he drank like a fish and smoked like a chimney. Perhaps we can all cling to that!'

Ah yes, but Churchill surely broke all the moulds, I said, because he believed he could. He believed he was a Great Man. He was utterly confident of it. He had sensed his own Destiny since he was a boy.

'Ahh, now that's very interesting,' says Desmond. 'Greatness is a highly relevant factor. This is important because one of the curious things I've noticed is that people who are happy in their lives can tolerate obesity, and apparently defy some of the health risks. If you're as successful as Churchill, you don't have to be "great" – just content with your life. You can stand being overweight more than if you are unhappy.

'The doctors will tell you there is a rigid link between obesity and heart disease, stroke and so on... These statements are very, very dangerous and I'll tell you why. Being fat is linked in some people to other aspects of their lives, and it's those other aspects that may be related to the diseases.

'A lot of half-baked research these days says that if you take 100 obese people, they are more likely to get such and such ailments, but what they don't ask is what it was that made those 100 people obese in the first place. You could be obese because you are, for instance, a Tongan enjoying the "primitive high status" that comes with being fat in your culture, or you could be obese because you are miserable and comfort eating, with lots of other things going wrong for you, and that means you're eating for the worst reasons in life – because you're bored or unhappy or anxious... Or you could be obese because you have a successful, fulfilled life. You don't have to be Winston Churchill. You could be a happy grandmother with scores of grandchildren around you...you don't do very much now, you've become overweight, but you are perfectly at ease with life. Your life may have changed, but you are still getting your carnal pleasures, and they still make life worth living – fat or not.'

Carnal pleasures, I ask? Come again? I've got the picture so far. I'm a grandmother, fat and happy, relaxed with life and surrounded by my superfluity of grandchildren. I can see it now, we're all gathered around the piano, singing Christmas carols while my daughters-in-law are slaving away in the kitchen preparing a feast of turkey with all the trimmings... But quite where am I, at this grand old age, with blue-tinted hair and half-moon glasses, getting my carnal pleasures?

'Ah! Carnal pleasures are very, very important to man! It's an old-fashioned word, "carnal", meaning pleasures of the blood versus pleasures of the head, body versus brain. We only have a few: sex, eating, sleeping, drinking. The point about these sensuous or carnal pleasures is that they are precious and key to a happy life, and when you get older those pleasures tend to move from the bedroom to the kitchen. I *am* speaking as an octogenarian! So what happens is that you can be perfectly content with your life, and your carnal pleasures are now taken at the table: you enjoy your food, and you can go to the supermarket and choose from thousands of different types.

'Such a person is quite different from the person who is eating out of misery and boredom, and the two should be separated in any statistic – they are not the same thing. But the majority of obese people today are, I think, those who are eating for the wrong reason – for comfort. One of the awful things about that is that there's no solution. It is no good telling those people to diet, because their obese habits are saving them...getting them through a really rotten time. That is something we all need to understand.

'What leads to their ailments is, I think, as much to do with their misery and anxiety as it is to do with their overeating because anxiety lowers the efficiency of the immune system. If you are fat and anxious, your anxiety is due to dissatisfaction with the way you are living, or the deal that life has handed to you – your family, your job, all of those elements. If you then suffer a heart attack, that heart attack was probably brought on as much by the misery as by the layers of fat on your body.

> *It's your lifestyle and your mindset that shapes your body and your health, not your diet.*

Fat and evolution

OK, so now we're back to the crucial question again: what makes the Naked Ape obese? Why should boredom, misery, dissatisfaction and the negative aspects of 21st-century life manifest themselves in fat?

'Let's start at the beginning,' says Desmond, settling into his armchair, and I'm delighted to feel one of his 'talks' coming on. This is better than any old episode of *Zoo Time*.

'The human species evolved primarily as an omnivore hunter-gatherer, which meant that our species was subjected – probably for about a million years – to an alternating regime of famine and feast. That alternation, caused by successful hunts, unsuccessful hunts, prey animals moving away, more prey animals arriving, meant that during the famine periods it was essential for humans to have some kind of fall-back to get through a famine.

'If you look at a monkey, it doesn't have the adipose fat layer that we have – it has loose skin. We have the adipose fat layer with the skin attached to it – it is a basic anatomical difference between us and our relatives; the chimp doesn't have it either. Uniquely amongst primates, we developed this layer of fat all over our bodies. And because in the early stages women were much more important than men reproductively, and had to be much more resistant to the famine period because they were rearing offspring, evolution produced a much heavier fat layer in females than males. That's why women have curvier bodies than men. Women have twice as much fat as men, and men have twice as much muscle. That difference is clear in the shape of the bodies. It also means that when there is too much fat, the woman will get fatter all over. In males, on the other hand, the fat layer is more like that of a camel with a hump – the fat is put around the belly, the pot-belly – and that develops on the male while the rest of him remains comparatively slim. It's a completely different pattern of obesity in the two genders.

'Now this system worked perfectly well provided you had these alternating periods of feast and famine. But with a supermarket, you have no famine periods. In the West today what you have is feast and feast, not feast and famine. No famine to knock off the fat. So if modern man is going to the supermarket every week to buy food, it's as though that individual has had a successful kill every week!

❝ In evolutionary terms, obesity will occur wherever, in the post-agricultural age, a culture is successful enough not to go hungry. ❞

So our bodies were designed for periods of plenty followed erratically by periods of near-starvation, and neolithic struggles of hunting and gathering in difficult environments. We still have that same prehistoric physiology, and it cannot cope with a supermarket culture.

But, astonishingly, it isn't just the abundance of food nowadays that's making us fat, nor even the domestication of our food supplies through farming. Desmond Morris believes there's more to it than that:

'We also have increased food variety, flavour and texture. We've improved all those things as part of our gourmet lives, and in so doing have made food much tastier, much more desirable, so that we are not eating because we are hungry – we're eating as a form of art appreciation.'

Art appreciation?

'Well, cooking is an art, and just as we like to look at paintings or listen to music, when we are eating today we are taking part in an artistic event. Feeding has become an art form, therefore the pleasures of enjoying that art form have gone way beyond diet.

'Two main factors, then – first, the loss of the famine/feast alternation, and second that we have now improved the taste and texture and variety of food to the point that it becomes an aesthetic activity rather than basic sustenance. Those are undoubtedly the factors that lead to the possibility of an obese culture.

'There are also genetic factors, I'm sure. Whether or not there are specific obesity genes, there are certainly activity genes, energy genes, because some people are driven and others are not. Some of us seem to put on weight very easily, others eat like horses and are stick-thin throughout their lives – and don't we all hate them!'

And yet, if it's all an accident of birth, or at least genetic inheritance, why are we as a society so unkind to fatties, so intolerant of obesity?

'Ah, that's because we don't look at the cause. We don't ask, "Is this person eating because they really love their food and are having a wonderful time eating it, are becoming connoisseurs and are very happy?" Instead we wonder if we are looking at someone who is comfort eating because they are miserable. We need to learn to think it through. If the majority of obesity is caused by boredom, anxiety or feelings of inadequacy, and our society is fast becoming fat, then the real problem is not the obesity, but the underlying causes.'

And how do you deal with that?

'That is where politicians don't understand human behaviour. One prime minister said to me, "Politics is simply to do with one thing: controlling inflation – that's all it's about; everything else is secondary." As Keepers, they tend to think that if you keep the cage clean and put pellets of food in, that's enough, they'll be happy...but that's not the way human beings are. Humans need excitement, variety, challenges.

'Life has lost all its risks – and I cannot help but blame this "health and safety" society we have created. Health and safety restrictions should be limited to things like dangerous door handles and dodgy electrical wiring, not to things like playing conkers and school outings into the mountains. If you take away minor risk-taking, like climbing trees or jumping rivers, perhaps, tragically, one child out of 10 million gets drowned, but the rest benefit from all the excitement of walking along a wall or jumping a river. If life loses all its risks, we suffer as a species, and that is what's happening now.

'There are how many of us on the planet now? Seven billion? But how many people can enjoy the varied, challenging existence that our ancestors enjoyed? The people who painted Lascaux [the caves in southwest France covered with stone age paintings] and made stone tools – they had huge challenges in their lives, and they did have to face famine from time to time. It was a challenging era – it went on for a million years – during which time you only succeeded if you had courage and imagination and excitement and risk-taking. That's what forged the species.

'The technological revolution of the past 30–40 years has suddenly removed a lot of the physical effort and activity, and it's produced a large population of which only a small percentage can enjoy the sort of challenges that our species likes to enjoy. If you have a life without challenges, you tend to switch off.

'Nowadays, even if you do want to take risks, you are stopped. Health and safety rules and regulations are contributing to obesity because they are stopping people from adrenalising. It is so sad. We actually need challenges to be fully alive.'

So it's not that we, as a species, have suddenly become lazy, I ask.

'Laziness is not a natural human quality,' asserts Desmond firmly. 'As a species, we have a very high level of curiosity, a very high level of playfulness, a very high level of energy – otherwise we would still be sitting in little tribes. You just cannot explain civilisation without that.

'If people have become lazy, it's because they haven't been given the joy of creativity, of exploration, the challenge that the human brain is capable of and needs. The human brain is an extraordinary thing: it flourishes when it is given all sorts of challenges, but if your challenge is packing cardboard boxes every day or making rivets in a factory, this will not satisfy the human brain, and eventually it will protect itself by switching off, giving up, becoming lazy. If they [the under-challenged] can afford it, they'll get fat.

'The trick is for politicians to find some way in which to give people challenges they respect. It's a tough task, almost impossible. Human beings are essentially creative – either destructively or constructively.

'I look at how housing estates are designed and despair – because that is where a lot of the trouble starts. There's nothing there. Where are the go-kart tracks, where are the dance halls (or whatever is the modern equivalent)? There needs to be something for fun and excitement, and if all you've got is a pub, don't be surprised if people use it, perhaps too often.

'Our Keepers need to look at every housing estate in the country and see what they could add that would provide some sort of excitement or challenge. In Oxford we have a big fair that comes once a year, and all the young people go and clamber on these machines that throw them around in the air, and they pump lots of adrenalin and get lots of excitement. Then the fair goes away again for a whole year. I'm not suggesting a permanent funfair would do the trick, but you have to ask why do people go year after year? It's the stimulation. Ordinary life...school...doesn't give them anything approaching that level.

'Young males in particular need risk-taking. They need to be able to take challenges sometimes – mental or physical. People sneer at these *X Factor*-type shows on TV, but in a sense they do at least lay down a challenge. The pity of it is that there is one winner and everyone else gets kicked out. What you want is something where you can have a new competition, a new winner every five minutes. It should be possible to find some way in which young people could be given more challenges. The health and safety mentality is dangerous because it is killing that off. And look what results – amongst other symptoms, obesity.

'Obesity, in the vast majority of cases, is no one's personal fault, but it is most certainly their problem. It is a problem that has been put upon them by the structure of the society in which they live – which is at odds with the kind of animal they evolved to be.'

And at the moment, says Desmond, the only effective action to be taken is personal...self-help. It's no good looking out through our bars to the Keepers. They don't yet understand enough about it to figure out what to do. So we must find a strategy to put 'play' and 'challenge' back into our lives. Pump adrenalin, take risks, work at being content, keep busy and stimulated, and let the fat fall where it will. It might even fall off!

Desmond likes to quote Eubie Blake, a US jazz pianist, who said at his 100th birthday party: 'If I'd known I was gonna live this long, I'd have taken better care of myself.' The irony is that it was probably his *not* worrying about his health that enabled him to live that long, says Desmond.

'It seems that if you wish to live an unusually long life, you need to eat and drink what you fancy, keep as mobile as possible, have a lively interest in the world around you, avoid introspection and, above all, do not waste time worrying about your health.'

Desmond Morris has studied man for long enough to know. Those who end up in early graves include both the food fascists and the couch potatoes, he says. The trick must be to find health somewhere in between.

CHAPTER 4

THE FAT DIFFERENCE BETWEEN MEN AND WOMEN

✳

A top obesity specialist said something to me the other day that really shocked: 'When did you last see a fat old man?' I had to stop and think, and couldn't come up with an image. Not that I go around looking for fat old men. But, come to think about it, I haven't seen one recently.

'Mmm,' he sagely shook his head. 'That's because they are very, very rare. Didn't used to be. But they are nowadays. Fact is, if you are a very fat man, you don't live to be old.'

Can this really be true? I've checked it out with quite a few of the obesity experts I know here in the UK, and they all started nodding their heads and agreeing. Men have an especially tough time if they get obese, mainly because they will stay in denial for too long and fail to get help. But, ironically, if they *do* address their problem, it can be an easier fix.

Fat men are very different from fat women. For them, it's much easier to lose weight – yet another sign that God is a man. Or that Mother Nature had a one-track, dead-end mind. Let the women have the babies and then let their bodies go to hell.

It's now official: it's much easier for men to slim down than women – that's the verdict of one man who has devoted most of his career to helping men battle their beer bellies. He's Professor

Garry Egger, specialist in exercise and weight control at the Centre for Health Promotion and Research in Sydney, Australia. And he pulls no punches when it comes to weight loss; he even helped the former King of Tonga change his eating and get on a bike.

'Obese men and women are very different animals,' he says. 'I see so many women who go on a diet with their husbands and get depressed because their husbands lose so much more weight than them. They don't realise it's because they have a totally different physiology when it comes to fat storage: they need to eat much less than men, and they are genetically programmed to keep their fat at all costs. It's the reproductive imperative. Nature and evolution designed them to hold on to fat to sustain themselves through nine months of pregnancy. Their body won't give up that weight easily.'

The only problem with men, says Garry, is getting them to realise they have a problem in the first place.

'Too many men are in denial – they can't even see their belly or their man-breasts or their double chins. A man will look in the mirror and see Arnold Schwarzenegger! A woman will look in the mirror and see a big fat slob (even if she isn't), and then try to do something about it, but is limited by her physiology.

'Too many men don't see a problem until it is too late – until they have a heart attack. Then, once they come in the door, they're dead straightforward. They say, tell me what to do and I'll do it. You give them the tools and they'll do the job! It's almost like they want it all spelt out on a spreadsheet – you know, like an architect wants to see the project laid out in front of him. I like working with architects – they're good slimmers!'

But not enough men are getting the help they need, says Garry. Not enough of them want to know. Garry started his evangelical quest to reduce the male belly in Australia over 20 years ago with a programme called GutBusters. It got a lot of publicity, helped a few men, but nearly broke the bank for Garry. He sold it to Weight-Watchers, who tried to run it as a special programme for men, but eventually they admitted defeat and closed it down.

'I've gone broke three times on men's initiatives because you just cannot get them involved. Yet for the few individuals you can help, it is so successful!

Still Garry battles on. Now he runs Professor Trim's Weight Loss Program for Men on the Internet, and he works with the World Health Organisation on obesity projects in Australia and the South Pacific islands. His work in Nauru, one of the tiniest Pacific islands (once prosperous because the British mined phosphate there), has thrown up some stunning thoughts about obesity – more of that later.

But men on the Pacific islands have traditionally been big: 'Historically, men have needed to be bigger to be more powerful, so traditionally the Islanders have liked their men big,' says Garry. Which is perhaps why, in the 1970s, the King of Tonga was the biggest of all. Taufa'ahau Tupou IV, who weighed 31 stone, dominated the *Guinness Book of Records* in the 1970s for being the heaviest monarch in the world. But in the 1990s he was persuaded to lose some weight, and enthusiastically led his 180,000 subjects in a nationwide slimming and fitness campaign. In doing so, the king shed around 11 stone to reduce his weight to about 20 stone.

Garry worked with the king's nutritionist, and is commonly credited with getting the monarch slimmer, fitter and on to a bike.

'He was massive, and it was difficult for him to ride a bike, but he used to do it, right down the main street in the capital! He was so fat that he couldn't turn the handlebars, so when he got to the end of the street, he had to have a team of guards ready to bounce him around in the other direction.

'Most of the king's success was through a change of diet and attitude. The Tongans used to believe that big is better – it was ingrained in their society – you had to be big, that was the way you used to win wars. The king, though, had type 2 diabetes, right up until his death, but because he managed it by nutrition, he never took insulin, and that was a tremendous achievement.'

But in one regard at least, the king was typical of most lesser male mortals. Once he'd accepted he had a problem and set his mind to change, there was no stopping him.

Fat's favourite place

'Men store fat, rather like a spare packet of sandwiches, around the middle. It enables us to get through the next famine, if you like,' says Garry. 'And the fat that's stored around the middle is more dangerous, far more dangerous, but it's much easier to lose.

'So we've got everything in our favour and nothing against us in terms of losing weight, except to get a man to admit that he's got the problem in the first place – that's the hard part. And nobody in the world has been able to work out how to do that. Aussie men don't do diets. You go out and you drink and you buy big trousers to cover up the fact that you're getting fat. That's until the heart attack, or you suddenly find you've got diabetes or some such wake-up call – perhaps the wife leaving the bedroom, or even home. That's when men come to their senses.'

Getting men to face facts

The Australian situation holds true in the UK too. Jane deVille Almond has been trying to get men to see sense for years. She's a specialist independent nurse whom you might know better as the matron in Channel 4's *Diets That Time Forgot*. Her varied career has seen her setting up men's health clinics in the back of a barber's shop in Wolverhampton, in pub car parks and at motorway service stations. She's dynamic, forceful and what her fellow Midlanders might call 'gobby'. She can talk, and she can talk the right language to the right audience.

'To get the health message through to men you have to talk their language and go to where they hang out. Men are shy about health stuff. You have to lower their defences.'

So how did Jane get the men in the barbers even started?

'Well, Greg [the barber] and I would stand in the shop and start talking about someone we'd made up – all about his health, and how he'd gone to the doctor and had a lump or something. But we wouldn't finish the story. Then the guys who were having their hair cut – who'd all been eavesdropping – would come up later and ask for the rest of the story. And that's when I could get them talking about their own health, what was worrying them. Quite often they just needed someone to talk to. One in particular confessed that he'd had suicidal thoughts – nothing to do with his health or weight. He just needed to talk and couldn't with his mates or with his family. Do you know, over 42 per cent of the men I saw confessed that they had thought of taking their own life in the previous year.

'Outwardly a lot of men are self-confident, gruff, even aggressive. But so many are depressed and feeling that life is meaningless. We really have to address this. But when we're talking, that's when I can check up on any health problems that are worrying them, or say quite simply, "Look, mate, you really need to lose some weight and you'll feel so much better".'

But men like to feel they're in control. Anyone who's ever been married to one, or the mother of one, already knows that. Well, it's just the same with dieting. Jane deals with men's reluctance to accept help by putting them in the driving seat of their own weight-loss programme:

'Men are much more likely to comply with a regime that they themselves have helped work out. I did a feature with BBC's *The Money Programme* on Radio Four, and once we'd given them the lowdown on exercise and nutrition, we asked them to come up with their own little plan. To men it's all new and exciting, and if you can combine it with a bit of technology too, they respond well to that. They like competition, so we sorted them out into groups, and the competition worked.

'It's a completely different rationale from women's. Women know everything about dieting. They can tell you the calorie count of absolutely anything. Men, on the other hand, know bugger all.

'A lot of men don't realise that there is a health problem associated with being overweight or obese. They don't think, "I'm overweight – hey, that's going to put me at risk of heart disease or diabetes,"' says Jane. 'Which is often why you don't see men coming for help until they have already been diagnosed. It also doesn't occur to them – as it does to women – that fat might make them undesirable or unlovable.

'One of my clients, Dave, has lost 6 stone. At 60 he was told he had type 2 diabetes. He just said he'd always been big. I told him he didn't have to be – he could actually change things for himself. When we looked at his meals, he'd be having six or seven sausages with his mash – he had no idea that was too much and it was fattening. Men don't know about calories, whereas women go to bed dreaming of them. Men have to be told. But once they've learnt, they're off! They don't so often put their weight back on again like women because even if they do, they know they have the tools to put it right.'

Jane told me about the Naughty Table she has at one of her men's slimming clubs. Some of her dieters will swear that they've been eating healthily...

'After these guys had talked about the healthy meals they were eating or cooking, I'd ask to see what was in their bags. And they'd tip them out on to the table and there would be all these snacks and stuff – bottles of Lucozade, a couple of cans of Red Bull, energy bars – stuff they'd picked up from the motorway services. There would be more calories than their daily requirements just in their bags!'

At the start of one club Jane asked the men to categorise themselves into one of four groups: underweight, normal weight, overweight, or obese.

✳ 10 per cent of the truckers said they were obese, whereas in fact 78 per cent of them were.

✳ 100 per cent of the men underestimated their waist measurement, often by as much as 19 inches.

'The truth came as quite a shock to all of them,' says Jane. 'So many men just don't see the problem, even though it is staring them in the face.'

So why are men failing to get the message until it is rammed home? In the UK some 66 per cent of men are overweight and obese compared to 59 per cent of women. More women are obese than men, but more men are overweight *and* obese than women.

In the UK, as in Australia, the USA and all over the world, most health campaigns are aimed at women. Nowhere is there a slimming product targeted specifically at men – not even the most popular weight-loss drugs. In the NHS there are no male-led or male-driven weight-management campaigns, which basically means that men aren't accessing help – yet they need it more and would be better patients in that they would respond better. Even over-the-counter diet products aren't marketed to men. Not even SlimFast.

'Why would men want a strawberry milkshake?' laughs Jane. 'I have tried many men on the milkshakes, but most of them moan that they're far too sweet. Men are really the poor relations of the health campaigns and slimming programmes, yet they have the biggest problem. They're our men, for goodness sake, and it's like no one cares.'

IF HE THOUGHT POLITICS WAS TOUGH…

Just in case you still think he's a plonker, let me tell you, I think former deputy prime minister John Prescott has been very brave to confess in his larger-than-life autobiography that he has suffered from bulimia.

OK, many cynics reckon it was a cheap way to grab headlines and turn his book into a bestseller, But they underestimate the ferocity of the storm into which Prezza has just willingly steered. Because if he thought he got nasty headlines and malicious, snide comments from press and people for his politics, he ain't seen nothing yet.

For some reason, the media absolutely loathes fatties, and seems almost deliberately to misunderstand the issues.

The day the news broke, I heard Radio 4's Sue McGregor – an informed and intelligent person – comment: 'I don't mean this unkindly, but his fight with bulimia seems to have been one which he seems to have lost!' The audience at Broadcasting House guffawed. 'I thought bulimics were, some of them, unbearably thin, poor things!' she added.

Then someone else made a stupid comment about Prezza's two Jags being to blame for his obesity, and so started day after day of cheap shots at Prezza's expense in the newspapers, on TV and radio.

And who would believe there were so many hundreds of pictures of him stuffing his face! Here he was cradling an enormous packet of fish and chips; there he was biting into a pie. Here he was sitting at a banquet, knife and fork at the ready and napkin tucked into his collar; there he was nibbling a sausage roll while on the campaign trail. The picture editors had a never-ending supply. And the vocabulary, unacceptable for any other medical condition, was vicious – 'greedy', 'lardy', 'Fat boy' – and everywhere the inevitable question that is, in itself, a massive insult: 'Did Blair know he had left a sick man in charge?' The use of the word 'sick' is cynical. It is not a statement about health – it implies that a bulimic is mentally unstable and unable to do his job.

Bulimia and anorexia wreck lives – whether they affect painfully thin schoolgirls or middle-aged politicians. Are they just another aspect of the obesity epidemic we're trying to fight right across the world? Is over-eating, like anorexia and bulimia, an 'eating disorder'? I'd say yes. Are these conditions a sign of mental instability? As you cannot control your eating, and your obsession with food may actually be controlling you, does that mean you are mentally incapable of dealing with the rest of your life?

On my website, buddypower.net, we have hundreds of men and women who lead busy lives, juggling work with running homes and bringing up families. Many have big deal jobs, managing companies, people, money. Many are nurses! They might have weight problems, but they are not unhinged.

Eating disorders – and I include overeating in this – are thought to be a symptom of stress. Stress is clearly a 21st-century disease, and shows itself differently in different people. Some turn to drink or drugs, or compulsive shopping or gambling. Others, like John Prescott, turn to food – even when they've just got home from a five-course banquet in the City. Apparently, when his bulimia became known within his immediate circle of family and friends, one close aide told him to simply 'eat less'. Fat lot of help that was.

After much nagging from the wife, Prezza did eventually go to see the House of Commons doctor, who referred him to a specialist in eating disorders. He nearly turned tail when he saw the waiting room full of anxious young women. 'Luckily, none of them shopped me to the press,' he remarked.

That's the first thing I thought of too when I tried to seek medical help for my weight problem. I was terrified that someone would recognise me and tell the papers. In the end, that's exactly what happened. When I was nervously awaiting obesity surgery in a Belgian clinic, some fellow British sufferer decided to shop me to the Sunday papers, which is how my gastric band became a subject of public fascination rather than my own private worry.

Now if that's not stressful, tell me what is! It's one thing to have a weight problem, or a suspicion that you're out of control with your food intake, but it's quite another to face the contempt of the media. Yet I know a great many Fleet Street writers, photographers and editors, many of whom have weight problems, and even more who are alcoholics. I dread to think how many might have drug habits too. In the various broadcasting centres I've worked in, I have been only too aware of snorting going on in the loos, and performers who go in looking hangdog and miserable and, moments later, emerging wide-eyed and buzzing. But they're OK, you see, because their problem is hidden rather better than the fatty's, bulimic's or anorexic's.

As John Prescott has discovered, the media still thinks fat is funny, pathetic and worthy of ridicule and scorn. Years of political bear-baiting might have prepared him for malicious attacks, but this is so personal, it could send anyone right back to the biscuits and ice cream.

What's the solution?

The belly is the key, reckons Garry Egger in Australia. Even if it's not caused by beer drinking.

'I see the belly as the gateway to men's health. When it gets so big they can't ignore it, then they come and see me. Men aren't interested in anything that others can't see, so their heart, liver, kidneys, lungs don't bother them – until they start playing up of course. But I actually had one man break down in this group: he said, "No one helps me with my weight. There are all these women's weight-loss programmes, all these diets, but I've got this belly and I'm sick of my kids poking me in the gut and saying, 'When are you going to have the baby, Dad?' and all this stuff. Can you do something about that for me?"'

It was a cry from the heart that set Garry on a 20-year course of medical campaigning, and it's been a roller-coaster too, he admits, with so many men reluctant to listen. If only he could help with the belly, he thought, help get rid of the obvious problem, then he might be able to help men with their other health concerns too.

'I have this theory that we have grown up to think of ourselves as the stronger sex, so you never show the guy in the cave next to you that you have a weakness or he'll come over and bop you on the head and take everything you've got – your wife and kids and all your kangaroo skins! So you have to feign that you're well even when you're not.

'But men do really need help because they're dying seven or eight years earlier than women all over the world.

'Everybody thinks that men run society, so surely they must be look after themselves – but, you know, it's just not working out that way.'

So what does Garry do with the men who break the barrier and come to him for help?

'I don't use anything fancy with the men. It's always just about total lifestyle change – always a bit of everything. Meal replacements work with men; it seems to appeal to them psychologically. You can usually get 5 per cent of their excess waist off within about a month, and then they are spurred on to greater things, to learn what to do to change more. Ten years ago we used to say that quick weight loss was a bad weight loss, but we don't say that so much any more because a quick weight loss at the start can be a great incentive, provided it's got clinical back-up. If they're doing it on their own, then quick weight loss is followed by quick weight regain.

'Then you look at their environment – not just the society we're living in, but the man's micro-environment – what's in the house, the workplace, the school. Some of the men I work with individually, I have actually gone into their homes and through their fridges and cupboards, and said, "That's gotta go, put that somewhere else, put that up where you can't see it! Next time you go shopping, don't buy this, don't shop when you're hungry – so when you get hungry at 9 o'clock at night, there's nothing in the house to eat!"

'If they're beer drinkers, I tell them they can go on having a drink because there's nothing particularly fattening about alcohol. We in Australia were the first to make public the correct story about alcohol and body fat, i.e. that alcohol per se does not make you fat. No way is alcohol converted biochemically to fat in the body – the body has to get rid of it because it's toxic. It's what you have with the alcohol that's the problem – and that's usually high-fat snack foods or massive curries.'

Garry tells guys that they don't have a beer gut – it's a beer-and-peanuts gut, or a beer-and-chips gut. Without the food, the alcohol is not such an issue.

Both Garry in Oz and Jane in the UK are mines of facts and tips about food, eating, drinking and men with health problems:

DID YOU KNOW...?

✳ Salted peanuts have added palm oil (and therefore extra calories) to make the salt stick?

✳ Canned fish, such as tuna, is put in sunflower or peanut oil because all the valuable fish oils have been squeezed out for sale to pharmaceutical companies to turn into fish oil supplements?

✳ A pint of bitter is 50 calories more than a pint of mild. And a pint of Coke or ginger beer is more than either.

✳ Around 20 per cent of men don't know the name of their GP.

✳ Nearly 80 per cent of men don't know where their prostate is or what it does.

✳ Erectile dysfunction is very common among obese men, and there's an inverse association between testosterone levels and waist size. The bigger your waist, the lower your testosterone levels...

✳ Overweight men get fat tongues.

✳ A fat tongue and a fat belly quite often go together.

Er...what was that? Fat men get fat tongues?

Apparently so, and that's what causes them to snore, have trouble breathing at night, and eventually suffer from sleep apnoea – which is dangerous. Garry is adamant he's seen it time and again.

'Although I have had pathologists say they don't see this, it is well recorded that parts of the tongue do fatten up, and that then occludes the windpipe at night-time when you are on your back asleep.'

He says that air passes awkwardly across the base of the tongue to the windpipe, and that's when you hear that deep 'flappy' snoring sound at night. 'That's why, when men fatten up, one of the first signs of that fat is the snoring.' Even more interestingly, there's a 'snoring weight'.

'If you can get a man down to a certain weight – and it's not necessarily his ideal weight – the snoring stops. Three or four weeks
into a weight-loss programme I get a phone call from the wife saying, "Hey, I've moved back into the bedroom!"'

So for obese men it's a sorry tale – more snoring, less sex. No
wonder their partners are dragging them to the doctor's door. So
here's the expert advice for men to take away...

KEY POINTS TO REMEMBER

✳ It's the waist size that's important. If yours is over 40 inches, you
need to reduce it.

✳ Admit your problem to yourself and take action.

✳ That fat stored around your middle is the most dangerous sort but
it's much easier to lose than weight elsewhere.

✳ Getting rid of your gut (losing weight) will help your mental outlook.

✳ Little changes make huge differences. A 5–10 per cent reduction in
weight can result in a 35 per cent decrease in health risk.

✳ Things won't just get better naturally. In fact as you age, the energy
required to keep your body alive – your metabolic rate – decreases at
around 2 per cent per decade. This means that by 60, you're burning
up about 10 per cent less energy than when you were 20.

✳ Abdominal fat, or a pot-belly, leads to a range of diseases, including heart disease, type 2 diabetes, gallstones, gout and some forms of
cancer.

✳ Change your micro-environment – from the food in your fridge to
the activity in your day.

✳ One weight-loss plan does not fit all, so tailor your plan to suit you.
The professionals now recommend combining and matching strategies to the characteristics of the patient.

✳ Buy a bike – and use it. (Bikes have suddenly outsold cars for the first time ever in Australia.)

✳ Get a pedometer and challenge it.

✳ Mow the grass with a manual mower.

✳ Do some weight training – research suggests it's better than aerobic activity for men of a certain age.

✳ All successful strategies include some form of lifestyle change.

The central point of all this keeps coming back to haunt us, doesn't it? You *have* to achieve a change in your lifestyle – and, of course, it makes sense. It's your lifestyle that makes you fat. It's the world's lifestyle that is making the world fat. But if you change the micro-environment – your own kitchen, eating habits and daily routine – and you can reverse the trend.

Although fat clearly affects men and women differently, we do generally like living together. All my experts agree that men and women who 'lifestyle change' together, stay together, and they have the best chance of preventing obesity happening to their kids. Something to think about over tonight's TV dinner.

BILL CLINTON AND CHILDHOOD OBESITY

*

We may think we have a problem here in the UK, but the USA is so scared of childhood obesity that it's brought out the Big Guns to fight it. And there's none bigger than former President Bill Clinton.

Yes, Bill Clinton, the workaholic, cigar-smoking, super-sizing president, who allegedly insisted on a Burger King chef aboard *Air Force One*, and finished every meal with ice cream, pie and maple syrup, and was even well known by restaurateurs for being a customer who 'cleans his plate'.

But now he's changed... He's thinner, his hair is white but still boyishly thick, and he proudly reckons he's the same weight as when he was a grinning Rhodes Scholar at Oxford, way back in 1968. What changed everything?

'The brush with death I had maybe had the biggest impact of all,' Clinton said, referring to his quadruple heart bypass surgery in 2004. 'I realized that one more time I've been given another chance, and I wanted to make the most of it.' (Gupta 2005a)

It seems strange, and desperately ironic, to hear this from a man whose charisma and allure to women has even got him into impeachable trouble at times. Because he says he was the 'classic fat band boy' as a child. At 13, he says, he was 5 feet 8 inches, weighed over 13 stone and was 'hardly popular with the girls'!

'I was fat for most of my childhood, and I hated it,' he recalls. (Gupta 2005b)

And that's what makes him such a potent figure now in the fight against childhood obesity. Because he speaks from the heart, and is determined that his post-presidential legacy will be to halt and then reverse the horrifying trend in American kids' obesity. He says that young people entering their teens have got to understand that whatever they do now will come to haunt them when they're 50. Kids born in this decade, he says, are developing diabetes at the rate of one in three – and that's why a massive campaign must start now. For the first time ever, he claims, a new generation of children in America would live shorter lives than their parents.

'That's immoral,' he has said on TV and in print. 'Just what sort of parents do we want to be?'

When Bill Clinton was a kid, his grandparents, who brought him up, piled his plate high with everything fried – and then poured gravy all over it. For many people of his grandparents' generation, it was almost an act of love to stuff food into children. Chubby babies were adored – their roundness was a sign that they were loved. My own mum recalls putting an extra spoonful of baby formula into the bottle – she says that all mums did it be-cause there was almost a competition between them at the baby clinic to see whose baby had put on the most weight!

Clinton recalls in his autobiography that a kid in the southern states (he was brought up in Arkansas) enjoyed a standard diet of fried chicken, cheeseburgers, fried ribs and chicken enchiladas, barbecue, potato salad, cinnamon rolls and sweet potato pie – all extremely high in fat and sugar – and he loved them all. On top of that, he recalls, he got little exercise.

That very childhood is possibly what makes his speeches such a powerful warning siren for today's children. No one stopped to think then that what he calls 'the aggregate' of too much fatty, sugary food and too little exercise would one day cause dangerous heart problems. But the former president is living proof that bad habits, built up over a lifetime, can suddenly sit up and bite you – often when least expected.

While he was in the White House, he was often lampooned for his inability to resist fatty fast food, though he was also well known for taking a daily run. He was pictured in a tracksuit and trainers many times, surrounded by special agents who'd had to do the run with him, often in the dark hours of the morning. Since leaving office, however, he has admitted in many interviews that, despite the daily run and the semblance of healthy living, he was still not eating a sensible balanced diet. Without that daily run, he has later admitted, he would have shown much earlier symptoms of the heart problems that were to follow his exit from power. He also blamed his heart problems in part on genetics – there is a history of heart disease in his mother's family – but admitted too that he might well have contributed by being too careless about what he ate.

What he didn't realise was that his arteries were more than 90 per cent blocked, which put him at risk of a massive heart attack. Alongside that, his cholesterol levels were very high and his blood pressure was going through the roof. His final presidential physical put his weight at 15 stone, his cholesterol level at 233 (5.9 on the UK scale), and his blood pressure at 136 over 84. After it was published, he joked to reporters that he ate too much Christmas dessert because it was his last Christmas in the White House and he wanted to enjoy it. Just three years later he was lying in an operating theatre, undergoing quadruple heart bypass surgery.

He told later how he'd been planning to join his wife, Hillary (then a New York senator), at the New York state fair, when he felt severe chest pains which at first he mistook for signs of exhaustion. But those pains were the harbinger of something far more serious. It wasn't a heart attack per se: an angiogram, in which dye is injected into the bloodstream to determine whether arteries have narrowed, showed that there were serious blockages – up to 90 per cent in two arteries. He admitted he was a heart attack waiting to happen.

The doctors wouldn't even let him go home from the hospital that day. Instead, like any other patient, he was kept in his room, and spent what was America's Labor Day weekend surrounded by family and friends, watching hospital TV. Reporters clamoured outside the hospital entrance, anxious for news. One enterprising photographer from a New York tabloid managed to sneak a long-lens snap of the former president on his hospital bed, playing the word game Boggle.

The next day, while most Americans enjoyed a public holiday, surgeons sawed his chest open, stopped his heart for 73 minutes, put him on a heart-lung machine, then relocated a vein from his leg and rerouted an artery from his chest to bypass his four blocked arteries. Clinton later claimed to have had what might have been a near-death experience, seeing circles of light and friendly faces flying off into bright lights.

Hillary told reporters she and daughter Chelsea had been as nervous as any relatives might be: 'Bill, Chelsea and I stayed up pretty late last night talking, playing games and just being with each other,' she said. 'These past few days have been quite an emotional roller-coaster for us.'

While the world waited to see if a much-loved and demonstrably human former president would fully recover, Clinton was sure of one thing – being 'given another chance' meant he now had to make a difference.

After the op...

Following his recovery from surgery, the American Heart Association approached him, wondering if he would be willing to campaign on 'healthier heart' issues. He went one better and decided to work with them, but focusing mainly on kids. Having been an overweight child himself, and having been shocked by the increasing incidence of type 2 diabetes among young children, he decided upon a new initiative that would help America's kids.

Meanwhile, he quickly changed his own lifestyle. First of all, he went on the South Beach diet and lost at least 20 lb, and now works out several mornings a week with a personal trainer. He takes time out to do at least an hour of walking every day, and takes more rest at night. He also insists he hasn't touched a calorie of junk food since his surgery. Not one – though he does still crave cheeseburgers and steaks!

Now he's determined to change the lifestyle of a whole generation of kids – and he knows it's a Big Ask. His William J. Clinton Foundation (that's what young presidents always do, apparently – set up a foundation to do good works – after all, he was only 55 when he retired) joined up with the American Heart Association to form the Alliance for a Healthier Generation. Its mission – to lead a huge counter-cultural movement to save a whole generation.

At the beginning he was asked – by some very thin TV reporters – whether obesity was a fitting subject for a former president. He replied forcefully that he was already working on tsunami relief and Aids, but cardiovascular disease, as the number one killer in America, deserved even greater and more immediate attention. He pointed out that obesity and diabetes were the main risk factors, along with smoking. Why would he not wish to get involved?

Clinton is adamant that there's 'no bad guy' in this story: he points out that it's our environment, changing work habits and sedentary lifestyle that are to blame, not individuals. Statistically, half of the American food dollar is spent eating out, half of that at fast food places, and more and more schools are struggling to produce nutritious meals because of financial pressures, with little nutritional education taking place. Most alarming of all, he says, is the rise in type 2 diabetes – the sort that used to be known as 'adult onset' diabetes, but which is now appearing in children as young as eight.

The facts were forewarned in a World Health Organisation report a few years ago. In the USA it was noted that up to 45 per cent of children with newly diagnosed diabetes had type 2, and most were overweight or obese at diagnosis. It is sounding alarm bells the world over. Because type 2 diabetes, particularly if developed when young, can wreck lives. (WHO 1997)

'We've got too many kids too overweight,' says Clinton, 'and they're walking time bombs.' (Gupta 2005a)

The diabetes bombshell

But what exactly is so devastating about type 2 diabetes, especially when it affects children? Brace yourself... It took a no-nonsense, hard-talking Australian to spell it out. When you hear his words, you might wonder, as I did, why we don't have nightly health warnings on television.

❝ Diabetes can make men impotent. And if a boy gets type 2 diabetes before puberty, as so many are because of obesity, he will probably be impotent in adult life. ❞

Just imagine a TV ad with that message. It should be on every evening around suppertime – just before *EastEnders* or during the *Coronation Street* commercial break: 'If he's your son, he might never know the joy of having his own children. If he's your son, you might not get grandchildren.'

It won't be a very welcome message in living rooms up and down the land, particularly if little Johnnie, sitting on the sofa with his supper on his lap, waiting for his favourite soap, is a bit tubby around the middle. But perhaps we need such a hard-hitting message for it to sink in.

Professor Garry Egger, *the* men's health expert in Australia, said it on national radio one day, and the station's phone system crashed under a huge barrage of calls from worried mothers and grandmothers. 'We'd never had a reaction like it!' he recalls. 'I've been going on about the dangers of obesity and diabetes for years, but when I spelt it out like that I was besieged by a whole generation of Australian women anxious that they weren't going to have grandchildren.'

It's true. Diabetes is a potentially devastating disease, which is tragic enough in adults, but it's absolutely appalling in children because it means that their bodies may never have the chance to develop properly.

'It is so shocking that you could say type 2 diabetes is nature's way of controlling the population,' says Garry. '[The disease] makes you impotent – and I had to say it. Next day – and I have never seen such a quick reaction – the Health Department rang me and said they wanted to put on a special conference because of public pressure – all within a day of that show going to air.

'It's incredible. Obesity itself gets no reaction, no sympathy. People don't really think about it – not even if you say it can cause early death. But to say a kid could grow up impotent, that got reaction.'

All the world experts I have spoken to agree. But little is known about the way type 2 diabetes becomes worse over time in children because, until recently, so few children had the disease. This means I can't give you any figures for the risk factor because there aren't any available yet.

As Bill Clinton says, type 2 used to be called 'late onset' diabetes because older people tended to develop it when their active lives started to slow down, and perhaps they didn't eat as well as they once did. Now it is becoming more and more common in pre-pubescent children.

Diabetes experts believe that the disease probably progresses just as it does in adults, gradually causing damage to the eyes, kidneys, heart, blood vessels and nerves. A child who develops type 2 diabetes may have an increased risk of complications in later life because he or she will have had the disease for such a long time.

Childhood – lost and found

The emergence of type 2 diabetes in childhood is a serious development. But so is the loss of a quality childhood. In San Francisco I attended the annual conference of the American Bariatric Association, where I heard a Brazilian surgeon talk about his latest case study on a group of morbidly obese children from São Paulo, one of the country's poorest cities. He said these kids, ranging in age from 12 to 16, were referred to him because they could barely walk. Most of them, he said, had been obese their whole lives, so they had never run around the school playground without being taunted and teased. They had never joined in football games because they simply couldn't keep up. They had never climbed on apparatus or swung from ropes, and were all too big to fit on swings – even when they were toddlers. Quite simply, he told a packed conference, they had no childhood. They were isolated and depressed.

He said the most noticeable thing about these kids was that they believed they were lazy and stupid. Everyone had told them so for the whole of their young lives. Their self-esteem was at rock bottom, which made them very difficult to help, so convinced were they that their predicament was all their fault and that they were completely beyond help.

They had been referred to him, a surgeon, because everything else had failed. He was given approval to operate on them – and he gave them all gastric bypasses. The change, apparently, was dramatic – and not just concerning their fat, which dropped off quickly. They started to move. They started to run and play, and even joined in football games. And they were shocked to find that they were *not* lazy. In fact, they enjoyed exercise and activity. They were like little animals unleashed from a cage. They were neither lazy nor stupid – and they weren't that different from any other children. Something had just gone very wrong for them from a very early age.

So why is this happening to our children– and who is to blame? If you let your child get that fat – no matter what your own problems are – aren't you effectively guilty of child abuse?

CHAPTER 5

FAT KIDS MAKE
FAT ADULTS

✳

The only effective way to beat obesity is never to get fat in the first place. Not even as a child. Once you've put on a lot of weight, you will never stop fighting it. Even if you do manage to lose weight, it will be a daily battle to keep it off. You'll never be able to relax your guard. Once you have been obese, your body will always act like an obese body. It will resist all your attempts to shake it off.

Many people, even if they manage to lose weight, might still feel they're fat *in their head,* and could be confused or unhappy – even with their dream body. There's no end to the struggle. Rather like someone who has abused alcohol in the past can never really shake off the demon, and has to accept they're an alcoholic for the rest of their life, if you've been obese as an adult or a kid, you are a fattie for life.

That's the real picture being painted by the world's top scientists – and they know that it's not very helpful, but it is the stark truth. Depressing, ain't it? The more I went to the top experts, and the more I met and interviewed obesity specialists around the world, the more it became clear. For anyone overweight and wanting to lose it, their message was the same. Fat is the Moriarty to your Sherlock Holmes, the Master to your Doctor, the Joker to your

Batman, the Green Goblin to your Spiderman, the Lex Luther to your Superman – the villain who can be defeated only by self-sacrifice, excessive discipline and dogged dedication.

Mother Nature never knew, when she hard-wired us for survival at all costs, that we would one day invent a world where food was abundant and inertia was a lifestyle. She gave us a body that was designed *not* to slim down. Mother Nature thinks fat is pretty good. It'll see you through the tough times; it means you'll survive to bring up the little 'uns, feed 'em with milk, and then who cares? The species has survived! (And, let's face it, Mother Nature has never really cared about us women in our later years. Be grateful you're allowed to sit in an armchair and knit.)

Does science hold the answer?

Scientists have given us the diagnosis. So can they give us the solution too?

I have faith in science. My dad was a scientist – a physicist. At least two of my sons are too. I grew up in a world dominated by equations and funny little pencil drawings of quantum theory diagrams on random sheets of squared paper – and my dad used to cut fruit in quadrants and feed us thin little slices that he called 'slivers of excellence'. Science was *all* in my childhood. (If I had my life over again, I would study physics just to please him. But, alas, I became a teenage girl and hell bent on everything but.) As a result, I was brought up believing that one day we will indeed colonise the moon and Mars, we will wear silvery leotards, pink luminescent wigs and Velcro slippers to counteract negative gravity. I was mortally disappointed that it hadn't happened by the 1980s because I was ready for it! I still am. My kids know that even if I am 80 and it is possible for tourists to fly to the moon, they are obligated to buy me a ticket! Even if they think I am totally past it. I want to see the good Earth from orbit. I only wish my dad could have done so. My sisters and I made sure he flew supersonic – we got tickets for Mum and Dad to fly on Concorde. But oh, my God, would he have loved to have soared in space!

I trust that science will provide an answer to this awful human problem of obesity. Just as I believe that if they put enough human energy, faith and money into science, physicists will come up with multiple solutions to global warming – without us having to totally abandon our comfortable and enjoyable lifestyles. Just look at cars. I'm already driving a hybrid, which saves money and energy. Why isn't everyone doing it? Give our scientists the right scope and they *will* find a way.

I respect Mother Nature, but I also trust science to find a solution. Not a get-out, not an antidote, but a solution to a major health crisis. I have to – because no one (except the scientists) will.

So the only glimmer of hope for an increasingly fat population will have to be provided by scientists. They are working now on a daily injection that will help us to regulate our weight in much the same way that people pop pills for high cholesterol or blood pressure. And there won't be any sense of blame about it, or of moral weakness or laziness or sloth. It'll just be something most of us will have to do in order to live healthily in today's environment.

'Is this the way society should go? I am not sure that's the question,' says Professor Jane Wardle at the Health Behaviour Research Centre in London's University College. 'It'll be just the same as people with high cholesterol taking statins,' she says. 'Do we make moral judgements about them? Or do we just accept that they have a problem and we know how to help them manage it?

'Perhaps one day there *will* be a pill that will treat obesity, help people control their weight and fight the adverse effects of environmental factors. It wouldn't be a cop-out or a quick fix, but a medical treatment. I'd love to be able to prescribe it and help people change their lives for the better just like that. But I'm afraid it isn't even a glimmer on the horizon as yet...'

Now Professor Wardle knows her stuff. She's not only a scientist, she's a medical doctor and a psychologist. She's studied the body and the mind, and how they interact. She looks at our behaviours and how they influence our health. She's so good at it that she's working with Cancer Research UK and finding out new ways of helping people to help themselves lead healthier lives – including how to beat cancer, reduce their risks of heart disease, diabetes, stroke...you name it. Her studies embrace everything and everyone, from babies to adults, thin people to fatties, genes to habits, nature to nurture. And, clever as she is, she's still learning stuff that will help all of us beat disease and conditions that affect all our lives.

She invites me to a cup of water and a coffee in what looks like a dingy office block just south of the great University College Hospital in Gower Street, London. It's summer and it's hot. Her office is adjacent to a coffee shop and one block up from a branch of Habitat. I'm shown in by a porter, who says I should go to the second floor. I feel guilty taking the lift. I am interviewing this tip-top professor about obesity, and really I should be bouncing up the stairs and arriving breathless yet glowing under a moist halo. I see no stairs, so I press the button and wait for the ping.

Professor Wardle is smiley and very slim. One might almost say thin. But I can't hold that against her just because I'm here to talk about fat. She's draped in a white linen dress, cool as a cucumber, but friendly and kind. I think if I was one of her fat subjects (for one of her studies), I might be daunted or put off because she couldn't possibly understand what it's like to fight fat! Yet I immediately like her. She listens. This woman understands. The compassion is in her eyes, her hand movements, her vocabulary – but particularly her observations. It's when she expresses empathy with the women who pushed fish and chips through the school railings to their kids that she really captured my attention...

Do you remember? When TV chef and food campaigner Jamie Oliver had made a huge impact on the school meals debate? And everyone was trying to do something about school dinners? That was such a brave move. After all, he could have sat back on his luxury livelihood advertising Sainsbury's lamb's lettuce and fettuccini, and made a fortune out of sugar, cream and fat, as so many celebrity chefs have done in the past, literally living on the fat of the land. (Oh, how annoying it is to see a chef making money out of simply pouring more cream on to a dish, or more sugar, or alcohol, or salt! We could all camouflage lacklustre cooking with such devices. I could do that, you must have thought!) Yet Jamie was uniquely brave, as perhaps only a very young and rich man can be. He spoke out. It made him notorious. It made him an easy target. And it made him very, very famous. Because basically, he was right.

Our school meals were, by and large, garbage. I know – I've seen 'em up close and felt both revolted and ashamed that my kids were expected to eat them. What was the budget? In some areas, it's less than 41 pence per child per meal. Dickens would be turning in his grave.

Personally, I think Jamie Oliver deserves a knighthood for doing what no one else seemed powerful enough, or brave enough, to do. He asked a very basic question: why are we feeding our kids meals that we wouldn't stomach ourselves? And he stuck with it.

Now, after individual schools, and even the government, had tried to 'up' the standards, we got one set of parents who seemed to be revolting.

'Pupils at a South Yorkshire school are being fed fish and chips through the gates by parents who say the canteen is not providing what their children want,' ran the local BBC news bulletin.

And there followed news footage of mums doing just that – driving to Chubby's the chippy with a huge list of take-away orders, buying armfuls of battered sausages, chicken and chips, packing them into plastic crates, then serving wrapped meals through the bars of the school's back fence, from the adjacent cemetery. I remember watching with mouth wide open – and not because I was salivating. I nearly threw my pizza wheel at the telly. It looked like crack peddling, like these mums were smuggling death and destruction, disease and decay to innocent schoolchildren.

What's a mum to do?

It all started, apparently, because the school , under the guidance of Jamie Oliver, revolutionised its school meals service and started to serve healthy options, restricting chips to Fridays only. Without consulting parents. Clearly many of the kids, and a few highly vocal and determined mums, weren't impressed.

'We're just giving the kids what they want,' protested one. 'The reason we have done this is because our kids are being served up disgusting, overpriced rabbit food by the school and are not allowed out at lunchtimes to buy something they can enjoy. Food is cheaper and better at the local takeaways. We don't make a penny on it. We just want to make sure the kids are properly fed. They don't enjoy the low-fat stuff at school, and the end result is that they are starving.

'Kids need a bit of fat in their diet – there is nothing wrong with burgers and chips. At school they only get chips once a week if they are lucky. The school have objected to what we are doing and they have even threatened to call in the police. But we will carry on.'

It made the national news that night, and was all over the next day's papers. It was immediately seen as a slap in the face for 'Saint' Jamie:

'Oliver's plan fails as pupils snub healthy school meals,' said the *Independent*. 'Oliver thought his exposé had done the trick when curbs were introduced on school meals in September 2006. Out went Turkey Twizzlers and burgers and chips, to be replaced by pasta, fresh veg and fish. Schools were also ordered to ban fizzy drinks, sweets and chocolate, and serve fried food just twice a week. A £220m cash injection over three years was promised by the government.

'But the figures seem to show that the mothers of Rawmarsh Comprehensive School in Rotherham, South Yorkshire, who passed 60 portions of fish and chips, hamburgers and fizzy drinks for children through the railings in protest at the new menus last year, were speaking for children across Britain. Youngsters seem to be relying on cheap take-aways and snack food to get them through the day instead. Almost two-thirds of secondary school pupils are shunning school meals, and around 60 per cent of primary school pupils.' (Herbert 2007)

The *Sun* described the women as 'junk mothers' who exhibit 'the kind of feeble parenting that turns kids into fat, lethargic burger addicts in the first place'.

'Mrs Chips takes order for the school dinner run,' said the *Telegraph*, which quoted another irate mum having a go at our Jamie:

'I just don't like him and what he stands for. He is forcing our kids to become more picky about their food. Who does he think he is? He can feed whatever he wants to his kids, but he should realise that other parents think differently.'

And Oliver riposted: 'I've spent two years being PC about parents. It's kind of time to say if you're giving very young kids bottles and bottles of fizzy drink, you're a f***ing a***hole, you're a tosser. If you're giving bags of shitty sweets at that very young age, you're an idiot.'

The head teacher, John Lambert, was outraged by the mums' behaviour. He'd tried his level best to turn around the standards of his canteen – for this?

'I'm stunned,' he said. He looked it. 'What these women are doing is unbelievable. They are encouraging children whose parents give them money for a healthy, nutritious meal to spend it elsewhere.'

My phone started to ring at that point. Would I come on to radio this and tv talk show that to debate healthy eating and child obesity? Britain was in lynch mob mode, middle-class mothers and nutritionists seething with indignant rage. What could these monstrous mothers be thinking?

In weighed the children's minister, Kevin Brennan, calling for all secondary pupils to be locked inside school grounds at breaks and lunchtime to stop them spending their money on snacks with high levels of salt, sugar or fat.

Then, like a splash of paraffin to feed the flames, came the inevitable backlash – from supporters of the mums, and from other schoolkids throughout the UK. 'Sick bag food' – that's what they called their schools' healthy meals. The *Evening Standard* managed to find armies of Turkey Twizzler fans:

'Joanne, 14, a pupil at a large comprehensive in London, is sucking her Triple Power Push Pop as she explains to me why she insists on stuffing her mouth with such sweets.

'I don't buy any of the stuff in the canteen, it's disgusting,'she says. 'The drinks are vile – there's no sugar in them. And as for the food, well, it's all salads and vegetables and stuff – and I don't like that.

'So I stock up before school on crisps and lollipops and chews, then at lunchtime I go and eat them where none of them nosy teachers is looking.'

So there I was, on Radio Five, joining in the witch-hunt. It was outrageous, I said, for those mothers to undermine what the school was trying to do – what the country is trying to do – for kids' health. Also, what lesson are they teaching their kids? That the new food guidelines are wrong? That you should openly flout rules and do your own thing?

Oh yes, I was right there, at the front of the moral crusade. When I got home from the studio to a kitchen full of boys making their own dinner from a pound of mince, a tin of tomatoes and a handful of mushrooms and peppers, I remember feeling 'Thank goodness my kids aren't like that!' Then my eldest confessed to me that he regularly bought packets of crisps and chocolate bars on his way to the bus stop, and resold them for vast profit in the school playground.

'I don't eat that sort of crap!' he protested. And he meant it. He was the one who started the family boycott of McDonald's, KFC and Burger King several years ago – to massive complaint from my younger boys – until we all watched Morgan Spurlock's film *Super Size Me.* 'I just sell them!' he declared, as though that made it quite all right. 'It's amazing how much kids will pay for a

Crunchie or a packet of Walkers by the time it gets to 1 o'clock and they're starving!'

I put a stop to his little business scheme immediately, by the way. Or at least, I think I did. He's at university now and I doubt his fellow undergraduates provide such easy pickings.

POVERTY OR IGNORANCE?

A recent survey has found that 14 per cent of UK youngsters have never touched an apple, orange or a banana, despite knowing the 'five a day' message. Many of the kids supposed a healthy diet was about starving yourself.

The report also said that giving pupils fruit and vegetables at school often results in their getting less of them at home. How depressing is that?

What's even worse – many kids don't even know that chips are made from potatoes, and that potatoes are grown in the ground. Shown a pomegranate, many kids guessed it was a turnip. Is this poverty or blatant ignorance? Is this the result of poor parenting, or a society that has somehow come to expect its fruit shrink-wrapped and antiseptic?

Ministers are recommending that corner shops get government cash to sell more fruit and veg. Around 120 shopkeepers in the north-east are to get £800,000 in a trial scheme to buy lots of chiller cabinets to display fresh fruit and veggies prominently and in an appetising way. Five hundred stores in Scotland are already signed up. Some might say that this is a nanny state initiative. But perhaps we need a nanny every so often to show us the right way. Otherwise, when are we ever going to learn the difference between a turnip and a pomegranate, and all the goodness that lies within?

What happened to Jamie's plan?

Sadly for Jamie Oliver, schools up and down the country started to realise that while he was talking the talk, pupils and parents were walking away. To name but one, Warrington Borough Council's School Meals Catering Service reported the 'Jamie Oliver effect'.

'The infamous Jamie Oliver TV programme, *Jamie's School Dinners*, shown in February 2005, has unfortunately had a detrimental effect on school meal uptake. It is a fact that parents have lost confidence in school meals. National benchmarking data from school meal caterers has demonstrated a decrease in meal numbers between 10% and 15%. In some cases meal uptake has decreased by 26%. This has resulted in significant financial deficits.'

Two years later, in 2008, pupils were still shunning progress, and just 37 per cent of them at secondary schools and 43.6 per cent at primary are choosing school dinners – pretty short of the government's 52 per cent target. There were even reports from hospitals treating kids who'd 'done a Jamie' – legged it over the school fence and hurt themselves scrambling to the local take-away.

What on earth does this say about the healthy eating crusade? Maybe it was just downright bloody rude to try and change a nation's eating habits by locking our kids on school grounds and then force-feeding them with steamed fish and salad? Perhaps the so-called warring mums in the Battle of Rawmarsh School – that's mums Julie Critchlow, Sam Walker and Marie Hamshaw – deserved to be consulted before we sought to fundamentally change their kids' food?

There's no doubt that in our fight against the flab, too many dietitians, chefs and so-called slimming experts have patronisingly taken a 'my way or the highway' approach bordering on food fascism, and it really does stick in the gullet. That's what those mums were kicking against, I reckon. They would like to have been asked. After the stink, and when it had all blown over, they wanted to make one last point:

❝ It's not that we're against healthy food. We're against people changing the rules without even consulting us. ❞

Back at UCL, I'd have expected the neat and trim Professor Wardle, whose work is all about changing lifestyles to save lives, to condemn them as sinners and child abusers. But nothing like it. She entirely understands their motives.

'It wasn't a pretty sight, was it? To see those mums shoving fish and chips through the playground bars like feeding time at the zoo... But I don't think it proved that they were bad parents. It simply showed that they were worried their children were not going to get enough food to last them through the day. They were actually trying their damnedest to be good parents. I'm sure I would do the same thing.'

Really, I asked?

'Yes! I would feed my child through the school railings if I was convinced that he was not going to eat anything that the school served at lunch. I know what it's like to be the mother of a skinny child. You spend all your time worrying if they're getting enough. So if I had the added worry of knowing that he hated school food and would go hungry, then yes, I'd smuggle something into him.'

Controlling too little or too much?

Interestingly, Jane Wardle has done another of her studies on mums who are overweight or obese themselves and the way they feed their kids. It relates to another of those 'blame' issues in the big, fat culpability climate surrounding obesity.

You know how you see pictures of fat kids in newspaper stories about childhood obesity? You somehow look for a fat mum too, don't you? It's a common prejudice. If we see a fat kid, we immediately want to blame it on the 'fat' habits of his mum. But Professor Wardle's study shows that, if anything, fat mums feed their kids no differently from skinny mums. Except, perhaps, that they exert a little less control. They give their kids a little more choice – more say in what they eat.

'You could interpret that as derogating their duty, exerting slightly less control over their children's food intake. But what did stand out very clearly was the evidence that mums are most controlling over the eating habits of their skinny children. You see, uppermost in parents' minds is that their children shouldn't be too thin. It's hard-wired into their minds. They do a lot of thinking about what should be in their meals and lunch-boxes...they want to make sure their kids get through the day. We call it an "advance fuelling model"!

'The children that parents find difficult to feed are the ones that don't seem to have much of an appetite. They're always trying to get them to eat more, even if they have no appetite.'

I know what that's like. One of mine doesn't ever think about eating. If he's caught up in a new computer game, or even at school when there are lunchtime clubs and societies to keep him busy, he'll go all day without food. I have to cross-examine him when he gets home. Time and time again, his lunch-box comes home still unopened, full of healthy wholemeal rolls, chicken kebabs, tuna salad, grapes – and the odd Mini Roll! It's not that he didn't like it – he just forgot. Even at weekends, when he's at home all day, I keep having to remind him to eat. While I worry all the time whether he is getting enough food inside him, at the same time I envy him so much. If only *I* never thought about food! If that's a gene, can I have gene replacement therapy, please?

We all know Mother Nature programmed us to feed our kids. She also set us to worry more about our skinny kids. But if we have kids with great appetites – and even kids who are fat – she played another trick on our minds, which might have worked fine in pre-historic times...

'We see them as "easy" children,' says Jane Wardle. 'They're great. They are a joy to feed – and often they come back for seconds. We call it a "healthy appetite" and we don't see anything about it as negative.'

In fact, parents of obese children don't see it at all. If you tell them their kid is overweight, they call it puppy fat and wait for it to disappear on its own. But nowadays, puppy fat ain't what it used to be. Puberty doesn't stretch out puppy fat any more. Yikes! Yet another blow.

It seems that the fatness 11-year-olds have nowadays is a bit different from the puppy fat of yore. There's something a lot more permanent about it. Also, a child with puppy fat 20 or 30 years ago was much slimmer than a 'puppy fat' child today. In other words, what we'd have called puppy fat then is normal now. What we call puppy fat today could really be obesity and a potential lifelong problem. We've all got bigger, and we accept a bigger norm.

But wait for it – there's more. Thanks to vaccination pro-grammes, antibiotics and Calpol, our kids hardly have a day off school with illness. That's great, isn't it? No more months of con-valescing from whooping cough or scarlet fever. No more pasty faces or pockmarked bodies. Childhood is a breeze compared to what my generation of kids went through back in the 1950s and '60s! I remember spending days feeling ill, tucked under a candlewick bedspread on the downstairs sofa, recovering from measles or mumps, reading *Bunty* and listening to my mum cooking bangers and Smash in the kitchen.

Those days are long gone. Our kids are in school every day. 'Off-colour' means missing just one meal, and then they're right back to Technicolor again. But even that is making our kids fatter! Those illnesses always put us off our food. So did the high fever of less serious coughs, colds and flu viruses. You'd linger for days with just a bowl of soup to keep you going, whilst happily watching the rest of the family stuff their faces. But nowadays children don't even have to suffer overnight fevers. We spoon in the Calpol and other anti-fever, over-the-counter medicines and they're right as rain within hours, and asking for a chicken jalfrezi with extra poppadoms.

Those old periods of appetite loss all added up, and stopped children getting fat, according to Jane Wardle.

'Natural events in life, like childhood illness, may have put little brakes on weight gain. We didn't realise that, and, of course, improved paediatric health has been a godsend, but those little things don't happen any more and that's another reason why we see our children getting fatter.'

So the real problem, then, wasn't the mums with their fish and chips and battered sausages. Perhaps they shouldn't be lynched after all? No way. The mums weren't the problem. In fact, they were the ones who had already identified the real problem – and much quicker than the rest of us.

The real problem was their kids not wanting that 'healthy food' – not even touching it. Not only that, but the kids themselves reckoned another *huge* issue was the fact that lunchtimes had been made shorter, queues had become longer, and by the time you got your plate of curried lamb lasagne with-a-minimum-of-two-vegetables, there was no time to eat it.

Mums know. You don't win children over by lecturing, hectoring and bullying them to eat their broccoli. That brings back hideous memories of one primary school I attended for a short time, where I saw a classmate reduced to a blubbering wreck when she was kept behind in the dining hall at lunchtime and forced to eat her food. She sat for the rest of the afternoon, weeping in front of a plate of greasy lamb, flabby, overcooked carrots and congealed gravy, and that's where her parents picked her up at collection time. In those days, parents didn't really question what went on at school, so I don't think there was any fall-out from this situation as there would be nowadays. But my friend won the stand-off because she never ate that plate of food. She probably still doesn't touch lamb and carrots.

I told my own kids this story. They said it was a problem that came up all the time at school – food fights between pupils and teachers. But they had a neat way out of the predicament. 'You just throw up,' they said. 'Teachers never force you twice.'

The backlash brigade have a point. There are too many food fascists gaining ground. We can't force kids to eat healthily – it just won't work. It'll more likely drive them back to the chippy. Yet isn't it important that we do something about their eating habits? After all, we know for a fact that most schoolkids who are let out into town always end up buying food from local shops, mainly fizzy drinks, chocolate, sweets, crisps, cakes, biscuits and chips. They often consume their entire daily allowance of fat and sugar in one flying visit to the local take-away. Can we achieve change without being school meal fascists? Without the fear of inspectors rooting through their lunch-boxes and reprimanding us parents for packing a Kit-Kat or a Wagon Wheel for afters? Without the scary prospect of getting an extra school report at the end of every term, detailing what your child has eaten?

That's already going on at the Heywood Community High School in Lancashire. They spent £19,000 on a sophisticated biometric scanner that allows pupils to pay for their meals with a thumb-print, and their choice of food is scanned, recorded and reported. My God! Nineteen eighty-four is alive and well. Yet the headteacher, Mr Yates, is proud of it:

'As well as monitoring those pupils who consistently skip lunch, staff can use the device to pinpoint those children with the healthiest diets and award them prizes, and steer those feasting on burgers and chips every day towards healthier options.'

Can't those staff just use their eyes and talk to the pupils instead? In an ideal world of course it would be nice to think our kids are saying no to chips and yes to wholesome, balanced food plates at school every day – but let's live in the real world. They're kids.

Surely there's too much government double-think going on here. That school with the scanner should get on with its job of teaching the three Rs, and use a bit of cheap and easy common sense and human interaction in the dining hall. And spend £19,000 on better ingredients instead of scientific scrutiny.

For a government that's allegedly terrified of being seen to impose 'nanny state' legislation, the present one seems to have embraced a police state attitude to school meals. Jane Wardle thinks lunch-box policing won't work anyway. Using her years of research with parents and kids, she's advising the government on things that will and won't work in schools. Letters home, for example, about children's rating on the National Child Measurement Programme, will have to be incredibly tactfully worded so they don't arouse anger and hostility, yet sharp and clear enough to make a sore point.

'We did a trial run on letters home,' she says. 'Our letters were very non-critical, non-punitive. Some parents didn't quite twig what it was all about. But quite a lot of the parents did take up the offer of advice, and said they implemented it at home. It didn't have any effect on their children's weight, though!'

NATIONAL CHILD MEASUREMENT PROGRAMME

The Department of Health's National Child Measurement Programme started in 2006, and had been going only a year before discovering the shocking truth that nearly a quarter of all five-year-olds and a third of all 11-year-olds were already overweight or obese. Rates of obesity were worst in the northeast, the West Midlands and London. Over the year 2006–7 some 80 per cent of British children (that's 876,416 individuals) were measured by school nurses in around 14,000 primary schools, though parents were allowed to opt them out. According to Tam Fry of the Child Growth Foundation, data collection methods were so questionable that no one quite knows how many did opt out. This has proved controversial, since many experts thought the fattest kids were those whose parents were sensitive to possible criticism, and were therefore never measured.

During 2007–8 the measurement programme became more comprehensive, and parents received a letter about the results for their child, with advice on what they should do if their child is found to be overweight. The word 'obese' was not used.

Weighing and measuring children only at the start and end of their primary school careers isn't good enough, says Tam Fry. 'We've passed up the opportunity of monitoring the middle-school years, when the ravages of school dinners, tuck shops and vending machines start to take their toll. Remember that the UK has an obesity epidemic now partly because school growth checks have been ditched by the authorities for at least a generation. Consequently, they have failed to notice the insidious rise of weight in some of our children, and society is now paying the penalty.'

Many experts and commentators, including me, were worried that subjecting children to weighing and measuring at school might further stigmatise fat children, and even encourage bullying from others. Evidence so far suggests that this is not happening, and that most kids see it as just another boring school ritual. How parents reacted to the letters sent out towards the end of 2008 has yet to be researched, and may be a different story...

'Look, it's a mother's basic instinct to feed her child,' Jane Wardle continues. 'Her job is to make sure her kid will have enough energy to get through the day. Your big worry is that your child won't eat his lunch at all, so you pack in a Kit-Kat because then you know he will at least have something. If a lunch-box inspector takes that Kit-Kat away, you're going to be very anxious – and so is your child.

'Ban vending machines, yes – but you won't get much public support for banning junk food from lunch-boxes. It just plain won't work. Parents need a huge amount more help to inculcate good dietary habits in their kids. And schools need huge amounts more help and support to create environments where children can eat well and do lots of exercise...at least in primary school. I don't think the children themselves should have to think about it. They shouldn't have to take on this burden. As soon as they venture forth into the world (between about 10 and 14), they are making their own choices, and then they do need to learn what's best. That's when we need to give them the best information and labelling. But we cannot lock all the bad stuff away.'

The government's School Food Trust, which was started to improve the nutrition of *school* meals in the wake of Jamie Oliver's campaign, says lunch-boxes should be checked by teachers or dinner ladies. But it's only a guideline – and guidelines are interpreted differently by different schools. Some have a common-sense approach, while others take a sniffier modus operandi. Some ban chocolates and crisps and ask parents to sign up to a food contract. Some have no school dinners whatsoever and all kids take packed lunches. Others do the exact opposite – insisting that kids eat school dinners that always require a knife and fork. There are lots of schemes and initiatives, some cheap and cheerful, others expensive and complicated.

'There have been literally hundreds of different school interventions,' says Jane Wardle. 'Many are elaborate, well resourced and glossy...'

But have they done any good? Have they reversed or even halted the spread of childhood obesity? Have they achieved...anything?

'Zilch!' reports Jane. 'You can try to improve the school environment – healthier foods and more exercise – all of them good for us in all sorts of ways. But in terms of obesity, they've produced only tiny results. Not nearly enough to make a dent in the obesity stats. It is so, so difficult to make a difference. So far, no one in the world has cracked it.'

FAMILY INITIATIVE CAN OVERCOME DESPAIR

It's a sad fact that some kids are driven to the brink of suicide because of their obesity. Jonathan Scott, from Carlisle, was 15 and weighed about 19 stone when he was finally driven to the depths of despair. He'd been a fat kid his whole life, unable to run around in the playground, hating PE lessons, and feeling shunned and bullied by the cool set at school. What's more, he was dreading the thought of more teenage years feeling isolated and unattractive, particularly to girls. So returning home from school one afternoon, he raided the medicine cabinet for every type of pill there was, swiped a bottle of his dad's whiskey, and decided to take the lot.

'I was standing there with a fistful of pills in one hand and the whiskey in the other, and I was determined to end it all,' he told me, 10 years on but still near to tears at the memory. 'I thought that it would end my pain – I really thought that was the only way.'

But something stopped him. He thinks now it was the thought of hurting his mum and dad, and his older brother and younger sister. He loved them. He knew they loved him. And that's what made him put the pills and whiskey down, and instead cry into his pillow once more, as he did so many nights.

His utter misery about his weight was a secret he expertly kept from his family. His mum, Pauline, was convinced he was happy. 'He was always bright, clever and usually had a big smile on his face,' she says now, deeply upset at the thought that her son feels his childhood was 'wasted' through his obesity.

He had his own kitchen cupboard, crammed full with sweets, chocolate, crisps and his favourite chocolate puddings. 'I know some people always blame the mum, but he had his cupboard because it made him happy. I didn't see him as obese; I just loved him. I cooked healthy foods for all our meals – I thought that was enough. I wish I had been more aware at the time because I would have done anything to help him...'

The suicide bid was a turning point for Jonathan. He vowed he would never feel that low again, and asked his family to help him change his whole lifestyle. Mum, Dad and his siblings vowed they would all help to change the family's lifestyle, and support Jonathan in his seemingly impossible quest. His dad's friend offered to take him to his local bodybuilding gym, and Jonathan took his first 'baby steps' to getting his body in better shape. He never counted calories or stood on the scales. He knew his body was changing shape because his trousers kept getting looser and looser.

'I just started going to the gym once a week with this friend of Dad's, and I got inspired by the other men around me. It was a macho thing to do. I gradually got the feeling that I could really change my body – and I did!'

Just eight months later, Jonathan achieved what he now calls 'a healthy average body for my age'. That's when he thought, 'If I can do that – what could I achieve if I really work for it?' Eighteen months later, on Father's Day, he stood on stage at a national bodybuilding championship – tanned all over, bulging with muscles (and not an ounce of fat!) in his 'posing pouch' – in front of a minibus-load of his friends and family who'd travelled to London to see him compete.

'I didn't win or anything,' he laughs now. 'The important thing was that when I walked out on to that stage, I belonged. I had a body worthy of the business. I stood there and looked out at the audience and thought, "You can never possibly know how far I have come!"' Except that Jonathan does tell his story now – to other kids whose childhoods are also being wasted through obesity. He works as an ambassador for MEND, the national charity devoted to helping families beat obesity.

'Not everyone wants to go the gym every day; it was just my way out of my own personal problem,' he says. 'MEND works with families to find what will work for them – it could be anything from getting a dog and taking it for walks, to going swimming, dancing or joining local drama clubs or musical activities – anything to get kids and their families out of the house and having fun together.

'Turning your life around can be done, but you need the love and support of family and friends – then almost anything is possible!'

International initiatives

You win some, you lose some. That's the way it is with initiatives, but even if none of them makes dramatic improvements, perhaps their cumulative effect will change attitudes. Betty McBride, of the British Heart Foundation, thinks every effort, from every corner of the globe, will count.

'It's what public health campaigners are beginning to call the "swarm effect",' she tells me, sitting under a display of all of the hard-hitting posters and slogans she's used over the years to make people stop and think about what they're doing to themselves. 'Obesity is too huge a problem to be conquered by any one individual or any single campaign – but together, all these ideas will start to change people's lives.'

In China the government is imposing compulsory daily waltzing lessons in every school. They are reportedly determined to turn a generation of chubby cheeks into twinkletoes! Student waistlines have apparently expanded almost as fast as the Chinese economy. Clearly it makes for a good headline.

There's also a rumour that in Singapore, where 18-year-olds have to do two years' national service, the military won't let them back out into civilian life unless their waist measurement is under a certain figure.

In Somerville, a district of Boston, Massachusetts, they're even trying a whole town make-over. School lunches have been overhauled, with lots more fruit and veggies added. Restaurants have agreed to offer smaller portions and healthier kids' menus. They even got out and repainted crossings to encourage kids to walk or bike more. In fact, the whole city went on a diet and fitness programme, and researchers reckon it's working. Compared with other Boston districts, children's weights are going slowly down.

NEW YORK'S NEW IDEA

The Big Apple has always been famous for its street vendors, selling everything from hotdogs and hamburgers to pretzels and bagels. Well, now there's a new kid on the block, the Green Cart, which will sell only fresh fruit and veggies so that people can grab a healthy snack option for breakfast, lunch or on the way home.

There are now 500 Green Carts on the streets of New York and I think they're a brilliant idea. The scheme is the brainchild of Mayor Michael Bloomberg, who has been brave enough to actually enforce healthier habits, such as banning smoking in bars and cooking with trans fats in all restaurants. So far his ideas have worked well.

Are you listening, Boris?

In Puerto Rico, the state of their kids has been designated an 'island-wide emergency', and an $8 million programme called Puerto Rico in Shape was launched last year to hire physical trainers and nutritionists in each city and town.

In Tasmania, parents are up in arms, lobbying schools to ban homework – they're blaming it for causing obesity in their kids because it's stopping them from playing outside. More power to their elbow, say I. Homework is turning our kids into little adults, like workaholics who bring stuff home and work all night to the detriment of family life. Home time should be for tea, television and playing with your mates, not hours of study. Let's stop all homework and take school a bit slower: sit GCSEs at 17 and A-levels at 19, and take the pressure out of school life.

In Australia and Ireland, cycling groups are campaigning for cycling to become the solution. In Britain we've already seen the announcement of our first cycling city, Bristol, in a £100 million government scheme aimed at encouraging cycling by making it safer, easier and more attractive for kids and adults. York, Stoke, Blackpool, Cambridge, Chester, Colchester, Leighton Buzzard, Southend, Shrewsbury, Southport and Woking will be trying similar schemes. I live in Oxford, which is already a biking city, but my family and I witnessed an horrific accident between a cyclist and a car almost outside our front door. There's a lot of work to do before we'll feel safe taking to our bikes again.

In Kyoto, Nintendo is designing fitness video games designed to get the kids moving in front of the TV screen. Wii Fit is already proving a winner. Unlike most other computer games, which are so isolating, the Wii gets everyone physically playing together, madly waving arms and legs. The Wii Fit program, with its special platform, allows you to 'build' your own personal character so that it can monitor your progress. First, you choose a body shape, then a face, hair, specs and clothing. My little 'Mii' was a bouncy, pert brunette with a ponytail and a red trouser suit. But when I stood on the Wii board and it recorded my age and measured my weight, my slim little Mii suddenly ballooned. Now she's a tubby little brunette and she gets pink in the face after a few minutes' jogging!

I can see why some parents think it's a little harsh when their kids are told by some computer program they mistakenly thought was a game that they're overweight and need to smarten up. We're a society that's made a load of mistakes, but do we need to punish ourselves quite so much? Childhood obesity is such an emotive issue that we're almost bound to disagree about the way forward. It's such an important problem that there is a temptation to hurl blame at loving parents, talk of child abuse and taking children into care, when compassion, empathy and hands-on education might be more effective.

It must be exasperating for those at the front line – the Jamie Olivers, the head teachers, the doctors, dinner ladies and dietitians

– to have their wise words and actions so ignored and even resented. But they have to keep going because we'll never be able to make a difference at school without the parents on board. We must find ways to engage them – to appreciate that we're all in this together. The first job is to get them to understand how serious this all is.

KEY POINTS TO REMEMBER

✳ Puppy fat is a thing of the past.

✳ Puberty doesn't slim down a fat kid any more.

✳ If your kid is overweight or obese, he or she will probably be like that for life.

✳ If your kid is obese, he could develop type 2 diabetes – dangerous enough in itself, but with the added likelihood that it could make him impotent in later life.

✳ Those old childhood ailments are no longer there to help control children's weight.

✳ As a mum, you're programmed to feed, but don't abandon all control and let your kids please themselves.

✳ You might not be the best person to recognise if your child is overweight or obese. Mums often don't see it – that's part of their programming too.

✳ If you are overweight or obese yourself, think how wonderful it would be to give your child the gift of a slim, fit future.

As I said at the beginning of this chapter, once you put on weight, you carry it with you for the rest of your days. You live your life fighting it or suffering its consequences. And that's a rotten legacy to leave your kids.

VOICES AGAINST CHILD ABUSITY

*

Mums and dads, and sometimes grans and granddads, who let their kids get hugely fat should have their kids taken off them. That's the growing feeling among social workers and doctors in the UK, where obesity has played a significant part in at least 20 child protection cases in just one year.

'It's child abuse,' says Tam Fry of the Child Growth Foundation.

'It's child abuse,' says Rotherham GP Matt Capehorn of the National Obesity Forum.

'It's child abuse,' says MeMe Roth of the US group National Action Against Obesity.

And already motions have been tabled and, so far, defeated – first at the British Medical Association and later at the National Obesity Conference – to treat child obesity as a child protection issue, and to consider taking obese children into care rather than leaving them in the environment and with the adults who allowed them to grow so fat.

'It should be a punishable offence,' says Tam Fry. 'Very obese children are taking up NHS resources that should be used for legitimate purposes. Parents have got to be held accountable for overfeeding their children or letting their children become fat without taking action...

'We must safeguard the sort of children who have a BMI of 46, are unloved by their parents, ostracised by schoolmates and friend-less, and who finally contemplate suicide as their only alternative. We must protect the child locked in his bedroom, unable to move outside because of his fatness, who is going to suffocate at some stage from sleep apnoea. We must save all those kids who are so neglected and abused by parents who appear to have no brake whatsoever on what the child is consuming.

'If you accept that society must protect the child who is mal-nourished, how can you possibly deem a child at the other end of the spectrum is not also suffering from abuse?'

At the outset, Tam Fry accepted that his motion would prob-ably be defeated – and it was. At the National Obesity Confer-ence countless health professionals warned of the dangers of a Big Brother system dictating to parents how they should rear their children, and spoke of the contributing dynamics to many child-hood obesity cases – including family breakdown, parental depres-sion and just plain ignorance of obesity and its dangers.

'Why are we so squeamish about this issue?' Matt Capehorn asked me. 'I've seen children who cannot walk without a stick be-cause they are so fat. If we saw a child who is skin and bone dying from starvation and malnutrition, there would be outrage if we didn't take them into child protection. Surely a kid who is dying of obesity deserves the same standard of care?'

Already, from the top to the bottom of the UK, many children have been placed on 'at risk' registers or taken into care because of their weight. Last year Cumbria County Council removed an obese eight-year-old girl from her family.

The tabloid newspapers fed voraciously upon the images of grossly fat Connor McCreaddie, who weighed 14 stone at the age of eight, and Samantha Hames, who was also 14 stone at the age of nine. They were even warned to stop eating by another obese teenager, Natalie Cox, who's 25 stone at the age of 15, and who's now hoping six months at an American 'fat camp' will put her on the road to recovery.

'They're twice the weight I was at their age,' she said in the *Sun*. 'Imagine how much they'll weigh at my age if they carry on eating. They must do something about it now or end up like me.'

Samantha's mum, Angela Collins from Walton-on-Thames in Surrey, insists she's a good mum and tries to curb her daughter's eating. 'Nobody wants her to lose weight more than I do. It's agony seeing my daughter this size,' she told the press. 'People will look at us and assume we're lazy or we're not trying, but it's not true. Can you imagine how hurtful it is for a mother to be told they're harming their own child?'

Samantha, who, remember, is only nine, eats a 500-g bar of chocolate every day and is a UK dress size 18. She says she just can't resist chocolate.

'I know I'm addicted to it but it's so creamy and yummy that I can't stop eating it,' she said.

Well, I don't know about you, but that made my blood boil. And even if it isn't completely true (and I have learnt to be sceptical about stories in certain tabloids), if a child keeps eating chocolate even when a parent doesn't want her to, it's inexcusable and begs the question, 'Just who is in charge in that house?'

Fact – an obese child is already losing his or her childhood, and may die early unless someone in their household really takes charge of their eating.

Tam Fry is worried that a feeble response to the child obesity/child abuse debate will fail to halt the rise in childhood obesity.

'Young Connor McCreaddie was sent back to live at home under a special care package, and now there's a news blackout on his progress,' he says. 'I think he needed tougher intervention – and the news blackout makes me suspect that this care package is not working. After all, if he were losing weight and doing well, why would they be so secretive?'

Taking every obese kid into care is unworkable anyhow. There are 140,000 children in the UK who are 'significantly' obese. If only a fraction of them could ever be considered 'abused', taking them into specialist care could be unrealistically expensive.

The finger of blame in all this points unswervingly towards parents. Even if you accept the 'Foresight' report's description of obesity as 'a result of a biological vulnerability to a toxic environment' (which I do), surely the parent's prime responsibility is that very environment?

I am someone who has suffered from obesity. I have somehow fallen foul of the 'energy in, energy out' equation, and it would undoubtedly take me at least another decade to figure out quite where I went wrong. But I am fiercely vigilant of the environment I provide for my kids – everything from the contents of the fridge and the lock on the biscuit cupboard to the sports and activities we undertake as a family. I *have* taken them to junk food restaurants in the past. I've even been photographed doing it – back in the 1980s when no one batted an eyelid at feeding your kids occasionally with chicken nuggets. Things are different now – and have been for at least five years.

Why haven't parents got the message that, even if you have let your own body go to pot, you simply cannot allow it to happen to your offspring? It's like alcohol. You might have one or even two glasses of wine in the evening. But you don't let your kids drink alcohol. You know it's wrong – it's bad for them and you tell them so.

I don't quite know where, when or how our obesogenic environment turned us into a generation of lousy parents – but that's what seems to be happening. No one is saying it's easy to bring our kids up to ignore the glut of advertising, to withstand the lure of 24-hour TV and computer games, to say no to instant gratification in the form of sweets and fizzy drinks. (We may have trouble resisting the odd biscuit ourselves.) But surely if you can see that your own child is suffering, you take immediate action. Not when they're 15 and can go out and buy food themselves, but when they are nine years old and can still be dumped on the naughty step until they stop screaming.

Telling it straight

There's a very thin, militant mother in America who says parents of obese children are guilty of child abuse. She's MeMe Roth – a sort of Sarah Palin of obesity. She doesn't mince words, and she has an air of take-it-or-leave-it arrogance about her that has endeared her to the media every time there's a weight story to discuss.

She's declared war on Girl Scouts of America (because they sell $700 million-worth of cookies every year), she's denounced *American Idol* winner Jordin Sparks for being a bad role model (because she's outspokenly comfortable with being overweight and eating junk food), and she reckons Santa should slim down.

Get this – she's even started a campaign for all women to stay the same size as the day they were married. It's called the Wedding Gown Challenge. It 'encourages women to focus on being fit for life – maintaining a healthy body mass index – well before, during and long after their wedding day'. What bliss it must be, living in her ideal world.

MeMe is especially vitriolic about obese children – and particularly their mothers. Well, she says in explanation, women have a special responsibility.

'Women are at the centre of the obesity epidemic. More than 90 per cent of family food-buying decisions are made by women. A child of overweight parents is 15 times more likely to become overweight.'

In a world where obesity is spreading faster than hot butter, perhaps she has a point.

'One of our biggest catalogue companies now has plus size clothes for children. That should be sounding alarms all across our country – instead it is normalising the problem. We need to stop being so worried about pointing out that someone is overweight...'

And that's why she got so upset about Jordin Sparks, who is a very pretty and talented 17-year-old African-American girl with a size 12 (UK size 14) body – which actually makes her smaller than the average American woman (now a UK size 16).

'Look, we know that before she went on to *American Idol* she was a plus size model, and had gotten into the habit of saying "I'm just a big girl. I love junk food... pizza, pasta, steak, having two crème brûlées instead of one, and we should love ourselves!" And we should maybe love our curves like she says she loves her curves, but we don't want to give this message that it's OK to eat junk food all of the time.

'She was wearing plus size clothes at age 12. Outrage should be guided at the parents: she should not have a weight problem at such an early age.

'If we want to instil positive body image and avert any sort of eating disorder of either extreme, then we want to teach our kids from day one how to take care of themselves. That's really loving your body, not eating whatever you want, only occasionally exercising, and then saying the words "I love myself".

'We've gotten to the point...where we are normalising obesity. We're so used to seeing morbid obesity that when we see someone who's 10 or 20 pounds overweight, we think "Oh, that's fine". Well, it's not fine. An extra 10 or 20 pounds does actually increase your risk of disease or premature death.'

MeMe coined (and even trademarked) the phrase 'second-hand obesity'. She uses it to describe how fat parents often have fat children. She understands the genetic link, but reckons you've just got to fight harder to beat your genes.

'I come from a long line of obesity and I am a mother of two. I have to fight it. When most people are saying yes to Girl Scout cookies and to birthday cakes and French fries, I'm saying no thanks. Genetics determines how the fat will be stored, but genetics never made anyone drive to Dunkin Donuts.'

Heavyweight help

Bill Clinton blames both nature and nurture.

'Our kids are fat because they are eating more unhealthy foods and exercising less. And the foods they're eating have higher sugar and fat content. Who's responsible? We all are. Too many parents don't have enough time to prepare – or believe they can't afford – healthier foods. Too many schools have stopped physical education programmes, rely on vending machines with sugary treats to raise much-needed cash, and don't serve healthy meals in the cafeteria. And too few restaurants and fast-food outlets offer low-fat, low-salt and low-calorie meals. (Clinton 2005a)

'So what we need to do is not just offer healthier meals – we need to change the way we prepare a lot of these meals. We've got to cut down on the fat and sugar content of the food our children are eating, and the size of the portions, and get them to exercise a little more. We cut out 50, 60 calories a day – that's just maybe a couple of cookies, and they'll lose 20 pounds over a high school career.

'It's all about education and habits, and also about making it easier for working people. Motivating kids...that won't be easy. They need to be handled with care. Kids need to know it's important, but fitness can't be boring,' he says. 'There's no shame, there's no embarrassment. We have to let them know it's all good, but you have to do it.

'We can change. We used to cook everything in animal fats – then we were told that was unhealthy and we changed. Now we cook everything in trans fats. That is unhealthy and we have to change. But we can alter a whole society's attitudes and habits if we work together.

'Maybe you cannot stop a busy mom, with five kids in the back of the car, stopping at McDonald's on the way home from school or wherever. But you can change what is sold to her – and that can make a huge difference...'

His Alliance for a Healthier Generation has already made some astonishing achievements. It has targeted childhood obesity in four ways:

✳ Through schools (driving junk food out of vending machines, providing nutrition education, and getting daily activity back on the agenda).

✳ To kids themselves (teaming up with Nickelodeon and Fox TV, providing online games, encouraging youth activism, clubs and societies).

✳ Through healthcare (looking at early diagnosis and better treatments).

✳ Through industry (not demonising the food industry, but trying to change it. They're working with companies such as Coca-Cola, Cadbury Schweppes, Campbell Soup, Danone, Kraft Foods, Mars and PepsiCo, asking them to promote the consumption of fruits, vegetables, low-fat dairy products and lower-calorie drinks, in addition to portion control.)

The message is getting through, with over 90 per cent of American schools implementing at least one of the Alliance initiatives, such as new menus and after-school or lunchtime physical activity programmes. The Alliance has signed up more than 30 companies and trade associations in the food industry to stop selling their products to schools, and to change what they do sell. Four states – Alabama, Mississippi, Oregon and Colorado – have enacted their guidelines into law.

They named September 'Go Healthy Month', culminating in a Worldwide Day of Play involving more than 850 events and attracting 250,000 kids to have fun and get active. And one of America's top celebrity chefs joined with the Alliance to provide recipes and tips that 'empower' kids and their families to develop a healthy relationship with food and cooking (www.healthiergeneration.org).

'We have to reduce the caloric intake – the number of calories people consume – and make the food better. And we have to have more calories burned by more exercise,' says Clinton. 'We're working with a neighbourhood group called KaBOOM! to build more neighbourhood recreational facilities, particularly in urban areas around the country. We're working with Nickelodeon, the kids' TV network, on something called the Let's Go Healthy Challenge. We've had hundreds of thousands of kids across America sign up. One young man who was about 80 pounds overweight is now about to do a kids' triathlon, and we see this happening everywhere.' (OGSC 2007)

It's all been going so well that Bill Clinton asked Arnold Schwarzenegger to get involved. You might expect Arnie – former bodybuilder, movie star and now governor of California – to be a great fan of fitness and healthy eating. And indeed he is. But, unlike Bill Clinton, he's a Republican – a free-market conservative who's rather against over-legislation. On the issue of obesity, however, he is determined, and has already made the harshest changes, banning all junk food and soft drinks from schools, and producing some of the best results.

'In California, of course, I have to say we are already way ahead of everyone else,' he proudly told a school that had just joined the programme and built a new gym and weight centre. 'For instance, we have passed tough laws to ban the sale of junk food and sodas in our schools; we're the only state that has done that. And we are adding more fruits and vegetables now, and wonderful lunches, healthy lunches, to our lunch programme. We are putting $40 million a year into physical education so we can hire more physical education teachers here in California. And last year we spent $500 million on arts, music and physical education, and most of that went to physical education so that every school has daily physical education activities, and so that we have enough PE teachers. I am very proud of what we have done.' (OGSC 2007)

So he might be. California was the 36th fattest state in the USA, but now it has dropped five places to 41st. (Colorado, by the way, is the nimblest, with an obesity rate of 16.9 per cent, and Mississippi is the fattest at 29.5. Where obesity rates are still soaring, it held almost steady. Mind you, not even a single US state is near the national goal of reducing the obesity rate to 15 per cent by 2010.)

Governor Schwarzenegger believes that the older generation is to blame for inflicting obesity upon kids today:

'There is a real obesity problem here in this state and in this country. It's an epidemic, and we have to do something about it. Physical education, of course, is an important component in that, exercising and diet and so on. And I'm sorry to say that it's our fault that so many kids got overweight, because in the '90s we cut a lot of the physical education programmes all over the country. And that has had a tremendous effect. In this last decade, Californians collectively gained 360 million pounds of bodyweight – think about that – 360 million pounds in the last 10 years... The average 10-year-old gained 10 pounds in this last 15 years. One out of three kids and one out of four teenagers are overweight or at risk, and that of course has a tremendous impact, because this leads to major medical problems like diabetes, heart disease, sleep disorders, depression, and it robs our kids of a healthy childhood.' (OGSC 2007)

So Arnie has issued a Governor's Challenge to all other state governors in the USA – to see if they can beat him in the fight against childhood obesity.

Rising to the challenge

Former Arkansas governor Mike Huckabee (you'll remember him – he nearly ran for president, until John McCain got the Republican ticket) could give him a run for his money. Literally. He took up running when his doctor scared him, by telling him he probably had only another 10 years to live. Problem was, he weighed 20 stone and had just developed type 2 diabetes.

'The doctor told me, "The way you are living, your stress levels, the kind of job that you do and your health situation, you may have 10 years left, and that is being optimistic",' Huckabee says. 'Frankly, I was facing the fact that I was in the last decade of my life – and I was only 48.' (Squires 2004)

He admits he was a chronic overeater who hated to exercise, but he reckons that alone should inspire many to lose weight –

along the lines of 'If I could do it, then anyone can!' As he puts it, 'I am just one beggar telling other beggars where to find bread.'

Huckabee's doctor initially advised him against taking any physical activity because his weight was likely to damage his knees. So he started walking.

'My first exercise routine was probably six minutes a day,' he says. But even that was a huge challenge. 'Walking a city block just about had me winded.' He gradually worked up to walking a mile and a half a day. 'Then one day I was walking and I thought, "This is kind of slow. Let's pick up the pace." And I was running. It just developed, you know, it wasn't a planned thing. Every step became its own reward.' (Squires 2004)

Now he's written a book to enthuse others. It's inspiringly called *Quit Digging Your Grave with a Knife and Fork*, a 12-step, no-nonsense programme to change your lifestyle. But the no-nonsense attitude did not go down too well with parents in his state when he passed a law forcing every child at school to have their BMI measured. Many saw it as an invasion of privacy. But Governor Huckabee went ahead with it anyway. (Huckabee 2005)

The small town of Arkadelphia was the first school district to take measurements. What it found was alarming: nearly half of its graduating children were overweight. One in four of the boys was obese. (Just think of the diabetes, and the risk of impotence!) The school sent letters home to the parents. Plenty of them weren't happy. But a lot of them did something about it. As one doctor put it:

'Many parents came to my surgery to discuss their letters. They said they hadn't thought their youngsters were overweight because they were the same as the other kids. And that's the problem – so many kids are overweight that it is becoming normal. Parents are in denial. Only the letter home got their attention that action was needed.'

As well as rapping parents on the knuckles, Governor Huckabee brought in legislation to improve school food and increase physical education, and to stop vending machines selling unhealthy snacks. In 2006 he proudly proclaimed: 'We have stopped the locomotive train of childhood obesity in its tracks. Now it's time to turn the train around and move full speed ahead to healthier living.'

Still, though, Arkansas is the seventh heaviest state in America – so there's a long way to go.

Unlike the UK, where most celebrities are still too ashamed even to mention the words 'overweight' or 'obese' – only Jamie Oliver has the courage to pop his head over the parapet, and politicians still seem to be in denial – America is bristling with famous faces at the battlefront, particularly where children are concerned. (Interestingly, they are all men.)

MeMe Roth, though, is worried about future administrations.

'Look who's at the table when it comes to discussions of child obesity,' she says. 'Just a couple weeks ago Barack Obama hosted PepsiCo boss Indra Nooyi as one of his economic advisers. And George Bush – to discuss predatory junk food marketing toward children – surrounded himself with Kellogg's, General Mills, Coca-Cola and, of course, Pepsi. This is like having a big tobacco company tell Obama, McCain and Bush how to handle kids and smoking. And nowhere in any of these discussions is the prospect of a restriction of advertising to kids. The precedence of conflict of interest when it comes to our children's health must end now.

'Let's finally recognise obesity as abuse – abuse of our children, abuse of ourselves – and together take action against it.'

CHAPTER 6

THE PSYCHOLOGY
OF FAT

✳

You are what you eat? No, you are what you *think*! It's your brain, often working on an instinctive or subconscious level, that makes you fat, not the food itself. It's the brain that makes you reach out for a second helping even when you're not hungry, or a chocolate bar when you feel low. And, funnily enough, it's the brain that can be the last to accept your new figure, even when you have slimmed down and lost a load of weight.

The mind is possibly the most powerful ally, and also the most formidable enemy, when it comes to weight loss – all psychologists know it, all comfort eaters have learnt it the hard way. Yet every January, we as a society buy into the nonsense values of a slimming industry that hardly recognises the power of the mind. It just addresses food intake and calorie consumption as though mathematics was the answer.

So why is it that, even when you know deep down in your psyche that diets don't work and that they certainly don't work for you, you still grab at the next one that comes along?

I don't know about you, but I am still a sucker for a headline that screams: 'Lose a Stone in a Week!' or 'Drop a Dress Size Every Five Days!' or 'Two Weeks to Your Ultimate Beach Body' – and I have bought some crazy products in my time. Like the 'Tornado'

Diet, which consisted of some revolting powdered food supplement that you stirred into a glass of water and drank every morning. The tornado? Well, that was the rather pathetic battery-powered stirrer that you also paid for in the 'starter pack'. You can imagine how effective that was.

This reminds me of something else I wasted money on years ago – the Pedometer Diet. Every 2000 steps it told you that you could eat a chocolate bar that was made by the same manufacturer. For 10 quid! I think I bought it off one of those shopping channels, very late at night, when resistance was low and common sense already asleep. I don't remember making even the first 2000 steps – the chocolate bars were too revolting to be motivational!

> 'I was staying at my sister's in California, and fell for all the amazing stuff they sell at you on TV,' says one of the buddies, Aleysha, from BuddyPower.net. 'It was called the 24-Hour Hollywood Diet, and it said you could lose 5 lb in 24 hours just by drinking one bottle of their stuff. It called itself a "meal replacement" – and I suppose it was because you couldn't eat anything for 24 hours! It was murder. My sister and I were both starving, and the only reason we kept going for the full 24 hours is because we'd paid for the privilege – about $20! To be fair, we both lost 2 lb on the scales the next morning – until we had breakfast. One coffee and a bowl of cereal, and the 2 lb was right back on again. The only thing it proved was that there's no fool like an old dieting fool. So here I am, a couple of years later and still looking for the perfect diet!'

'Emma G' says her New Year's resolution every year is to use the mini-gym she bought from a slimming magazine to get slim and trim, instead of as a clothes horse in her kitchen.

'It's great for drying because it has so many bars and knobs and angles,' she blogged. 'But I could have bought a drier from Argos for 10 quid – instead this mini-gym cost me £300 and have I ever done anything with it? My husband keeps offering to sell it to one of his mates, but I won't let him because I swear one day I will use it properly. But I still haven't. Now I can't find the instructions, and I've lost the video that went with it!'

Mmm. Reminds me of the exercise bike gathering cobwebs at the back of my garage – and the hideous step machine lurking under my stairs. And didn't I buy a rowing machine once upon a time? Yes, I did – it's now languishing in my sister's attic!

Personal trainers and even equipment suppliers are now warning how much money can be wasted if you don't sort out your attitude and thought processes before spending up to £1000 on a bike, a treadmill or a mini trampoline. One top trainer told me: 'It's the New Year's resolution mentality, but it only lasts for a couple of days. People suddenly think they're going to run on a treadmill in their living room for an hour every day, but they haven't changed their mindset enough to change their routine. Exercise only works if you don't have to make a special effort to do it – it has to be part of your everyday life. That's why you get such great deals on second-hand treadmills with hardly a scratch on them! Good intentions aren't enough. You can't change your body if you haven't changed your mind.'

Mind your head

The power of the mind is a remarkable thing. Mindset can distort our perception of reality to an astonishing degree, as with anorexia sufferers who see themselves as fat when they are in fact emaciated.

I remember once taking the sort of dieting pills they don't allow nowadays – amphetamine derivatives, otherwise known as 'speed' – and still feeling a mysterious need to eat, even though I wasn't remotely hungry. The drugs acted on the hunger pangs, but not on the emotional craving. When I moaned about it to the doctor (a respectable practitioner at a Birmingham slimming clinic) he simply prescribed me some more pills. He never once remarked, 'Perhaps you aren't eating because you are hungry – perhaps you are eating for some other reason...'

For some slimmers, a trip to a psychologist or counsellor might be more appropriate than a prescription for pills, or even a diet and exercise regime. For bariatric surgery patients I strongly think a course of counselling should be included in the aftercare, which presently consists of merely dietary advice and one or two 'fills' (see page 24).

I have met gastric surgery patients who have lost a great deal of weight, but still feel fat in their mind. Take Francine Hodges, a middle-aged mum whose weight-loss story was featured on ITV's *Super Size Surgery*. Once 23½ stone, she had a gastric band operation and lost an astounding 14 stone. She is now petite and slender. If you met her, you would never imagine that she had ever been dangerously obese. Although the gastric band operation helped her to lose weight, it did not alter her mindset. Afterwards, instead of being elated at her new shape, she still 'felt fat' and was perplexed at the attitude of her family and friends, who wondered why she wasn't instantly happy. She still craved food for comfort. Her emotional needs still existed as strongly as they had before her operation, only now she couldn't comfort herself with food because the gastric band prevented it. The band physically stopped her from comfort eating, and thus highlighted what she believed to be an eating disorder.

'The band didn't fix my head,' she told me. 'When the weight start-ed coming off, I started to realise, "Hey, I am still wanting to feed something here!" and I started getting pissed off with the band and the way it was stopping me eating for comfort. I was contradicting myself all the time. On the one hand I was celebrating the fact that I could fit into slimmer clothes, but I still had this crazy head where I was sabotaging my band – trying to eat and then making myself sick... What I had was an eating disorder, but I didn't know it then. In fact, I always thought only skinny people had eating disorders. Now I know that many fat people have eating disorders too. And many have a sort of 'mid-life crisis' when they lose a lot of weight – it brings to the forefront of their minds a load more garbage.'

Other patients who become 'suddenly skinny' (a term now used on chat shows in the USA) through weight-loss surgery find that their new body fundamentally changes the family dynamic. Those who were happy with a fattie in the family now feel resentful, envious or displaced. Husbands feel threatened by a newly slim and attrac-tive wife. Wives worry that their newly lithe and youthful husbands may stray. Divorce is common in many an after-story.

Francine, who now coaches patients before and after surgery, says they rethink who they are and what they want, once they gain a new body.

'Many women, especially those who were fat their whole lives, go home and look at everything differently. They look at their grumpy old husband with his beer belly and his bad temper and they think, "Why am I putting up with this?" The truth is they always deserved better, but they put up with bad stuff because they didn't feel they deserved more, because they were fat. Now they've got higher self-esteem, they want more from life – and they go out and get it!'

Francine feels that people should understand before their operation that surgery, which can mean fast weight loss, has psychological side effects both good (as with enhanced self-esteem) and possibly bad. Because something new is coming to light. While it's openly discussed in the USA, I have found that few surgeons or clinicians in the UK want to acknowledge it. Yet again, it suggests that gastric bands and bypasses, as with pills, diets and exercise regimes, do not address the psychology of fat. I am not saying that everyone who is fat has a psychological problem, but clearly some people do. For them, as we shall see, it may be even more important to include counselling in their treatment.

Unwanted after-effects of surgery

I have met people who have experienced what is beginning to be dubbed 'addiction transfer'. This is when an addict is cut off from one addiction and takes up another. A food addict, for example, whose surgery physically prevents them from feeding their addiction, might turn to alcohol, drugs or even some other obsessive compulsive disorder.

Psychiatrists reckon that because weight-loss surgery has become more common – and patients more candid – they're seeing increased cases of alcoholism, obsessive shopping, compulsive gambling and even promiscuity.

Some women are turning to sex because, without food, they feel a distinct void in their lives. Now that they are slim, more self-confident and possibly more attractive to men, it follows that an affair is one way of trying to satisfy themselves. One woman described the feeling as 'an addiction to attention', and it drove her to have 14 affairs in all, including seven one-night stands, five of those with perfect strangers. One psychiatrist bluntly described this phenomenon to me at a surgery conference in America: 'After the euphoria of rapid weight loss fades, a harsh reality appears: life is still tough, even if you can fit in an airplane seat! Most obese people are emotional eaters, and when you take their food away, they're still left with those emotions.'

It could only happen in America, I thought. But I asked my friends on BuddyPower and I was staggered at just how many replied with real and heart-rending stories of addiction transfer, right here in ordinary homes in the UK. One of my buddies wrote:

'God help us all and shame on those money-making doctors who don't tell us that we may be trading one addiction for another. I was obese and miserable with many health problems, but nothing compares to being an alcoholic. I never dreamed in a million years it would ever happen to me. It has, but there is no surgery to cure this addiction.'

Another blogger from the USA says:

'My husband had bariatric surgery a few years ago. He weighed over 30 stone. Now he weighs less than 15. Before his surgery he could barely walk. Now he is fit. Before his surgery about all he could do was sit in front of the TV and eat. Now he can do anything he wants. Only now, about all he wants to do is sit in front of the TV and drink. It is simply a matter of watching the one you love step out of one prison and check into another. If you go through with the surgery, be prepared. You *will* be left with an emotional void clamouring to be fulfilled. You will have to choose your new obsession. I pray to God you choose something positive and constructive rather than falling back into a slightly modified version of the same trap.'

One emailer said she's an educational psychologist who works in public health, and she wants to campaign and raise awareness of this new side effect:

'I had my bypass in December of 2000. I was 21 stone and went down to 10. I have since gained back 4 stone, along with a full-blown alcohol addiction. Then my husband left, I lost my house, my job, my car, went bankrupt, and moved back in with my parents. I am literally having to start from scratch. My immediate interest is in getting gastric bypass physicians to deal with the "real" things that happen to patients as they start to lose the weight. The medical community is denying this problem with the alcohol and they will eventually get sued.'

Yet another correspondent wrote:

'I had gastric bypass surgery in August 2005. Since then, I've had a multitude of complications, with excessive drinking being one of them. I gained back over 2 stone and I'm now the same size I was before the surgery. I am embarrassed to let anyone know that I even had the surgery. I believe the reason I am not losing weight is because of my drinking. People think that surgery is the be all and end all – but they do not have a clue!'

One of my male buddies summed it up short and sharp:

'Five years out of surgery. Halved my weight! Last night I had 18 beers! I do have a drink problem now. I try to quit every Monday, but it has been two years now...'

Buddy Sarah, who has not had surgery, sympathises:

> 'I have found that since cutting back so much on food, I seem to want to drink miles more alcohol than before (or maybe I am just noticing it). I think it is a case of if I can't make myself happy by bingeing, then I will drink wine to compensate. The only way I am getting round this is by having decided to cut it out completely, which is not what I had hoped for, but it is seriously slowing my weight loss down.'

Real life

Possibly the most well-known addiction transfer patient is the singer Carnie Wilson, daughter of Beach Boys pop icon Brian Wilson, who became a singing star herself as part of Wilson Phillips. Carnie was 'the fat one' who eventually got pushed behind her slimmer co-stars. In fact, she weighed 21 stone and was regularly ridiculed on the American comedy show *Saturday Night Live*, and also by US shock jock Howard Stern.

Finally, she'd had enough, and after comedienne Roseanne Barr recommended it to her, Carnie opted for a gastric bypass in 1999. Amazingly, thousands of people watched her operation because it was broadcast live on the Internet. That operation saved her life and her health. Within the first eight weeks she had lost about 5 stone, and she dropped another 8 stone after eight months. 'It feels as if I blinked and the scale just went, "Whey"!' she told me when we met in San Francisco in 2007. 'It was the answer to all my dreams!'

For Carnie, a self-confessed emotional eater (she reckons she started as a child when her dad left home), it was the end of a nightmare existence, staggering from one diet to another, and always feeling like a failure. In 2003 she posed naked for *Playboy* magazine (with a teddy corset covering her surgical scars), and who could blame her?

Can you imagine, after a childhood and teenage years burdened by a shape she hated, what it must have been like to find she had a beautiful body worth flaunting? At the time, she said, the feeling of elation was almost intoxicating.

Sadly, though, Carnie's struggle was not over. Even with a gastric bypass, her weight started to increase again. She's even been on America's *Celebrity Fit Club* to try and lose the weight she'd regained. Worse, she became an alcoholic. She says she never drank much before her surgery, but afterwards she started drinking up to 10 margaritas a day, plus a bottle of wine in the evening. She was even drunk during the *Playboy* shoot.

She told Oprah on her *Suddenly Skinny* show: 'The drinking progressed more and more, and I found I was getting drunk very fast and I was getting sober very fast, and it was frightening because I saw myself going down a dark spiral very quickly.'

Carnie soon began waking up every day wondering how she was going to stop drinking. The stress of being known as 'the poster child for weight-loss surgery' only made things worse. 'I didn't want to be a failure,' Carnie says. 'And that gave me anxiety. And that made me drink.' Carnie reckons many people with weight problems actually have addictive personalities, as she does, though she doesn't blame the surgery for what happened to her. 'The weight-loss surgery didn't cause me to be an alcoholic,' Carnie says. 'I'm just a born addict.' That, she told me, is what keeps her campaigning and speaking out publicly about her problems.

We agreed that dangerously overweight people cannot wait to fix the problems in their head – the underlying reasons they are fat in the first place – because that could take 20 years. We both accept that surgery doesn't address your mental or emotional state, and that's why some forms of surgery don't seem to work for everyone.

What you need is aftercare that treats not just your physical needs, but your mental ones too. In other words, as Carnie puts it, 'weight loss now, therapy later'.

'You can't always solve it all before going under the knife because there just isn't time. But you should consider getting therapy later on, while you're losing weight and getting used to a new body.'

❬❬ Surgery doesn't fix your head. You cannot put a band around your brain, which is perhaps where you need it most! ❭❭

Get a strategy, not another addiction

We all have our own fears – our own no-go areas. Alcoholism is one of mine. My paternal grandfather ran a pub called The Diamond Bar in Greenock, on the river Clyde. According to my grandmother, he drank all the profits, then left her and their two sons to mop up the mess.

I have never drunk very much. I absolutely hate being out of control, and I find others' drunkenness really revolting. So when I heard about addiction transfer as a possible side effect of obesity surgery, I started to quake. What if, I thought, I develop an insatiable urge for alcohol once I can't eat much any more? After all, I already know I am an emotional eater. I just love spending 'me time' – not that I get much of it – curled up in front of the TV with a big plate of my favourite food and perhaps a small Bacardi and diet Coke. What if, as the plate of food got smaller, my Bacardi got bigger – what then? Would I do a Carnie?

So I took her advice and got me a course of cognitive behavioural therapy, or CBT, to address that very issue.

Cognitive behavioural therapy

CBT is the new buzzword in weight loss. It's about developing strategies that will help you. For instance, I have developed a totally new evening habit that will stop me ever developing an addiction transfer like Carnie's.

I have reasoned that I reach for a drink in the evening because I hit a chemical low. Often it is related to an emotion. Always it leads to me scoffing a bag of peanuts or some other snack and thinking, 'To hell with the diet today!' I don't need that snack, and later I will regret eating it, but that doesn't stop me.

A few years ago, when one of my children was at boarding school, I used to have to drive him back to school late on a Sunday night. By the time I reached home again, I would be feeling so low and drained that I always needed a drink. Often I'd pour it thinking: 'I've had a tough day. I'm tired. I deserve it!' Or sometimes it would just be a way of treating myself – a little luxury. I wasn't pouring a drink because I wanted a drink. I was reaching out for a comforting pat on the back, or a metaphorical hug.

So now, whenever I feel like that, I make myself a smoothie. Usually strawberry and banana, served in a gorgeous crystal cocktail glass. It's important that it feels as luxurious as possible – like a little taste of opulence. It reminds me of holidays in the Caribbean. Only 60 calories, and brimming with natural sugars and goodness. I sip it gently and feel almost immediately lifted. Ten minutes later I don't want or need an alcoholic drink – in fact, I've forgotten all about it.

It's a tiny, tiny strategy but it works for me. That's what CBT does – it teaches you how to strategise for better habits. Another simple strategy is to do something else with your hands – keep your fingers too busy to hold a chocolate bar or delve into a packet of crisps! To this end, PopCap Games, a worldwide computer gaming company, has actually funded research into what they call the 'possible therapeutic effects' of so-called 'casual' video games. This came about after discovering that their regular players said playing puzzle and word games, such as Bejeweled, Peggle and Bookworm, were helping them to lose weight. Was it just a coincidence? Was it because their fingers and brains were too nimble to nibble? Or could some games actually have a dampening effect on appetite?

A preliminary trial has suggested that they certainly do reduce stress levels and lift overall mood, but could we ever see computer games being prescribed for weight loss? Watch this space! A team at East Carolina University's Psychophysiology Laboratory is even now preparing clinical trials. Dr Carmen Russoniello, associate professor there, maintains that there could be 'a wide range of therapeutic applications of casual games' in mood-related disorders, such as depression, and in stress-related disorders, including diabetes and cardiovascular disease. In a stressful world we need all the help we can get, even if it comes from a small screen.

I reckon therapy or counselling should come as part of the aftercare package with any surgical procedure for weight loss. In fact, for many people, it may actually be a waste of time and money to undergo surgery without committing to counselling. It is every bit as important as the nutritional information and dietary advice.

So what is cognitive behavioural therapy? And why is it fast becoming the cornerstone of successful weight-loss programmes around the world?

In a self-help world, where there are thousands of books and videos that offer instructions on turning yourself into anything from a millionaire businessman to a great lover, you can also learn how to become your own weight-loss therapist. Even if you are already wedded to a diet that seems to be working for you, or you've had weight-loss surgery, you could still find it incredibly useful, and discover its effects influencing other areas of your life.

You don't have to be mad to do it! Neither do you have to endure months or years of regressing into your own childhood, or raking through the skeletons in your family closet. Although it does suggest that your problems are of your own making, it's not about self-blame – just recognition that sometimes we are our own worst enemy, and the way we think could be bringing us down.

CBT, recommended by NHS Direct and sparingly available on the NHS, is used for treating all kinds of problems, including obsessive compulsive disorder, anxiety and phobias, post-traumatic stress, depression, anger, habits (such as facial tics), drug and alcohol abuse, eating disorders, relationship difficulties and sleep problems. It's even used to treat people with arthritis and irritable bowel syndrome, the idea being that while it can't treat the symptoms, it can help people to develop coping strategies.

It is, as you might well have worked out, a mixture of cognitive therapy (which looks at our thought processes and why we think what we think) and behavioural therapy (which is about making deliberate changes to habits and reactions). CBT links the two together and gives the 'patient' a step-by-step programme to follow, learn and practise. In every case it is unique and tailor-made to the individual.

This form of therapy is pretty highly thought of, and I have met several slimmers on the brink of surgery who decided to have one more go at something else before taking the plunge. They opted for CBT and have managed at last to get a grip on their eating behaviours.

I decided to go and meet one of the first CBT therapists in the UK – American-born Kristina Downing-Orr. She's a lecturer at Oxford University, a broadcaster, clinical psychologist, author and journalist, and has even been a psychological commentator on TV's *Big Brother*.

'It all boils down to realising and understanding that we are self-medicating with food,' she says quite simply. 'It doesn't necessarily mean you have a huge psychological issue to address. It doesn't mean you are overweight or obese because there's something seriously wrong in your head. It probably just means that when you are under pressure, your coping mechanisms take you to food, and you end up in a cycle where you feel bad about yourself – you eat – and then you end up feeling bad about yourself again.'

Kristina reckons that a great many people are caught in that destructive cycle. 'And it is not easy to find your own way out. Often you need help from someone outside your circle of friends and family. That's because it may suit some of your friends, or even loved ones, to see you stay fat. Perhaps it makes them feel better if you are fatter than them. They may not even know they feel that way, so they are not being deliberately negative, obstructive or unkind. But they are still sabotaging your efforts by telling you that you don't need to slim, you look fine...'

I tell Kristina that there are hundreds of members on my Buddy Power website who complain of exactly that – friends and relatives who appear to be supportive but are actually bringing them down. One buddy wrote:

'I love my sister but I hate her as well. She's slim and she keeps telling me all I have to do is eat like she does. She offers to come and stay and cook for me. Every time I try to diet, and then fail, she tells me not to worry because my face is pretty and I can "get away with" the rest of my body. She even says it doesn't matter what I look like because I am a "lovely person". Everything she says sounds nice, but it's like there's a double meaning to what she says. It just makes me feel worse – and then I feel guilty for hating her!'

When I read that I actually felt sorry for both of them. When you are fat and hate yourself and your failures, not even a loving sister can say anything right. And the sister – well, she might be being catty, or she could well be trying to voice her non-judgemental support and be being unfairly judged herself!

'Sometimes even loved ones will sabotage you because your predicament makes them feel better, and this does happen a lot,' observes Kristina. 'Your action – going on a diet or joining a gym – may be threatening to them because if you are addressing your problems, they're thinking maybe they should address theirs! That's why people will sometimes try and talk you out of doing something about your weight – because then they don't have to address their own issues. No one acts and everyone's happy.'

Except, of course, they are not.

'There's something rather nasty in the human psyche that makes us feel better if we can look at others who are worse off than us – it's about competition. So often we need to look outside our closest support for real help and assistance.'

And that's where CBT comes in.

A typical CBT session

Kristina says: 'First, if someone came to me for help with their weight, I'd say, "Go to your GP". I'd want to make sure they are healthy, that there's no underlying medical cause. I'd recommend, "Go on a healthy diet, work with your GP," and only if they cannot stick to their diet or they find they're binge eating, particularly after a stressful event, then I'd say there might be some sort of psychological problem underpinning that behaviour – and CBT might help.

'You see, it's not an event that causes us stress – it's our beliefs about ourselves that cause distress. So, for instance, if you have a fight with your husband and then you binge on cream cakes because you are upset, it's not the fight that's triggering the eating, it's the emotions brought out by the fight. You might be thinking, "We're always fighting, we're never happy, he's always putting me down, I'll never be perfect..." All of these kinds of thoughts are flooding through your mind, and you turn to food perhaps because it makes you feel better and calms you down. So I always say to people – it's not the fight, or even your dissatisfaction with your own appearance that causes your overeating or binge eating, it's the belief about yourself that underpins that behaviour.'

So first you have to identify the belief and the trigger that causes it. A CBT therapist would recommend you to keep a food-and-mood diary or some kind of chart so that the next time you go into a binge-eating episode, you can write it down and see the connections for yourself.

'Say you are looking forward to going out Saturday night – to a party. And you try on the dress and the zipper won't do up. Now you write down in your diary: "I wanted to go to this party. I couldn't fit into this dress that I really wanted to wear. I was so upset that I raided the food cupboard." So I say, "OK, let's look at the reasons why you felt bad. Was it just because the dress didn't fit, or what you thought that said about you? What were those feelings that it brought out?" Usually they're feelings like "I looked so fat. I'm not attractive, that means I'm always going to be alone. I'm worthless. I'm morally bankrupt because I cannot be thin like all my friends."

'We really beat ourselves up with these emotions...and it's usually because we feel so bad, based on our beliefs, that we resort to binge-eating behaviour, and that just leads back into the cycle of feeling worse about ourselves. So the first thing you must do is find out what triggers the behaviour, then analyse the feelings themselves and then we work together on how to redress the balance...'

'So many people moan to me: "Yet again, I couldn't stick to the diet. It's the hundredth time I have tried, and I failed... I am such a failure..." So we need to examine all the reasons why people think they are a failure...and chances are, they are not a failure at all – it's just that in this one particular episode they have let themselves down, but that doesn't mean they cannot learn about themselves, learn how to take steps to improve.

'Once we tease out what that emotional factor is, we can start to build up that person's self-esteem and confidence so that the next time they cannot fit into the dress, they don't immediately go for the biscuit tin. They start to think: "What steps do I have to take to fit into the dress?" Or perhaps, "It isn't a tragedy if I have to buy a bigger dress...it's not the end of the world, it's OK – I'll get there if I want to get there, but if I don't get there quickly, then it's not a disaster, the world isn't going to fall apart. And it doesn't mean I am a complete failure.'

Is a therapist really necessary?

It seems so simple – and *is* so simple and logical – that you wonder why this message has to be delivered by a therapist at all. Why can't we figure it out for ourselves?

Kristina agrees – it *is* simple. But sometimes you can't counsel yourself; you need help, tuition, practice, coaching. The goal is a change of mindset, and that takes time and work.

'The idea is that instead of feeling failure and going to the biscuit tin, you learn a new reaction – you learn how to look at the reasons you feel bad, and learn how to take the steps to make yourself feel better...in a way that's not destructive, in a way that will no longer sabotage your goals.'

In a nutshell, then, it's the difference between 'I can't fit into this dress, I feel bad, I am going to eat biscuits' and 'I feel bad, I can't fit into this dress, but so what? I'm going out to see friends I like who don't care about how big I am, and I wouldn't want to be with people who are so shallow that they would judge me on my size anyway!' It's about figuring out your own values, living by them, and not living by the crazy values of others. They should teach it in schools, I reckon!'

Kristina says too many people indulge in self-destructive behaviour without realising it – binge eating is only the tip of the iceberg. She's seen clients who exercise too much, who spend hours in the gym, punishing themselves without realising why.

'Some people use food the way others would use alcohol or drugs, or spending, or gambling, or even exercising...as a coping mechanism because they are feeling bad about themselves. Once you realise that the behaviour is destructive, you are making the unconscious conscious, and you can then take steps to improve...'

Self-destructive behaviour, such as overeating, overspending or drinking too much, is usually secretive, says Kristina. 'The key is to ask yourself why you are hiding it away from others. You also have to ask yourself, "Am I overstepping the bounds of normal behaviour?" So many overeaters never eat in front of their families, and even their spouses have no idea how they could be so fat!

'People do feel the need to overeat when they don't really want to, but once they understand that there's some sort of emotional connection, then it's great to have the support of other people who understand because we are often surrounded by people who don't get us, don't understand the problems that we are experiencing. We all react to the pressures, stresses and events in life in different ways, and it's easier to speak to a stranger. Whether that's to your GP or a psychologist, or to support and self-help groups, it's important that you learn better coping mechanisms.'

CBT is generally a short course of therapy: '...you learn how to become your own therapist, you learn the tools you need to identify the triggers, to identify the underlying emotions that maintain your destructive behaviour, and find ways to cope and redress the balance so your behaviours become more beneficial. It takes eight to ten sessions, and once you get the principles, *you* take charge, and that is empowering in itself,' says Kristina. 'Your whole mindset changes, and even if it all seems quite simple, the results can be quite radical.'

I'll say! Since I started CBT, I've bought a bike and now regularly cycle around my village – because I like biking. I did it not for exercise, but for quality of life. Just doing that most mornings has put roses back into my cheeks and lost me another 6 lb of fat. I've become (slightly) more organised. I've taken up t'ai chi – just for fun. And I've got my old easel and brushes out and am painting again because I now know I need 'me time' that doesn't revolve around food. You can't nibble when you're painting – you get crumbs on your masterpiece!

Doesn't it make you think perhaps we shouldn't be so obsessed about weight, size and numbers on the scales? Perhaps we'd all be happier and healthier if we just concentrated on improving our quality of life?

LIFESTYLE INTERVENTION

The new buzzphrase in the war on fat is 'lifestyle intervention' – and it works, but it's expensive because it involves ordinary people needing expert, hands-on care for many months. Could we really afford enough lifestyle intervention clinics to help everyone who needs it

'Can we really afford not to?' asks Gary Frost, professor of nutrition and dietetics at Imperial College/Hammersmith Hospital, where the Fat Team also works. While other scientists try to find an answer to the fat problem with pills, gene research, hormone injections and the like, Gary's team is trying to find out if lifestyle change could be the better key – even if it involves what the NHS calls an 'intensive management package'.

Gary's Lifestyle Clinic requires six months' dedication and commitment from each of his patients. You're given specific goals and targets, taught how to spot your own weaknesses, and coached to alter your perceptions about eating and taking exercise. You visit once a month, but are set a lot of homework in between times, with constant phone contact and check-ups. After six months they have seen some dramatic results, with patients losing many stones in weight *and* keeping it off. Here are some of Gary's expert hints and tips on lifestyle intervention:

✳ Keep a food-and-mood diary, recording every morsel that passes your lips and your mood at the time. Write in a notebook that's small enough to fit in your pocket or handbag, and make it as vital to your everyday life as your wallet or your house keys.

✳ If you cut down on food, your metabolism will slow down a little. Don't let this happen – increase your activity.

✳ It doesn't have to be a punishing regime. An *extra* four three-minute walks every day will lose you 1 lb a month: over a year that adds up to almost a stone!

✳ Don't snack! A chocolate bar is 350 calories, but you'd need to walk briskly for an hour and a half to burn it off.

✳ Try to have meals of oily fish (such as mackerel, salmon, trout, sardines and fresh tuna) twice a week, and fill at least half of your plate with vegetables.

✳ Go for stronger, smellier cheeses – the powerful flavour means that you'll use less of them!

✳ Understand which are your trigger foods – these are the ones you feel compelled to eat whenever you see them, you find it hard to stop eating once you've started, you eat even when you're not hungry, and you eat instead of a meal. Then develop a coping strategy for them. For instance, try buying single chocolate bars instead of multipacks. Before you start to eat them, stop and think about how you're going to feel afterwards. Rate your hunger on a scale of 1–10. If it's less than 7, resolve that you won't eat.

✳ If stress is one of your triggers, go outdoors for 10 minutes and breathe fresh air. It will change your perspective.

✳ If you must have biscuits in the house, store them out of sight, or freeze them so you can't eat them immediately.

✳ Resolve to eat in only one room of the house, and do nothing else while eating – not even watching TV.

✳ Lapses are only human, but they don't come out of the blue – they are usually triggered by something, so find out what.

✳   Remember, it's what you do after a lapse that's most important. Don't let a lapse catapult you backwards. That's what the Fat Team calls catastrophising. Regain control.

✳   Beware hidden fats. We tend to judge food portion size by eye. But high-fat foods can contain double the amount of calories of high-carbohydrate foods, so know what you're eating.

✳   Avoid using your frying pan. Microwave, steam, poach, bake, boil or grill instead.

✳   Instead of crisps, chocolates and cakes, find alternatives quick fixes, such as yoghurt, crackers, rice cakes, fruit and raw veggies.

✳   Measure out oil rather than pouring it straight from the bottle.

✳   Use less meat in all dishes, and bulk out meals with extra veggies, potatoes and pulses such as peas, beans and lentils. Changing to more resistant starches, such as in lentils and pulses, could mean that less fat is likely to be laid down in the abdomen.

✳   Small changes make a big difference. Change your portion of fried rice to a bowl of boiled rice – that saves 200 calories. Change your daily full-fat pinta to semi-skimmed – that saves 175 calories. Change your morning elevenses from two chocolate chip cookies to a banana – that saves 65 calories.

✳   Remember the 10:10:6 rule for fat, sugar and fibre on food labels. These are listed per 100 grams, so look for foods with *less than 10 g of fat and sugar* and *more than 6 g of fibre*. (As for salt, aim for less than 0.1 g.)

✳ Not all nutrition labelling is what it seems. Remember, if it says '85% fat free', it means there are 15g of fat per 100g of food. Similarly, 'low fat' can often mean 'high sugar'.

✳ Eating out? Go for a starter instead of a main course. Opt for a broth rather than a 'cream of' soup. Have fruit or sorbet for pudding – and don't dip into the bread basket.

✳ When choosing ready-made sandwiches, look for packs containing less than 400 calories, or less than 20 g of fat for the whole sandwich. And don't reach for a packet of crisps to go with it – get used to a piece of fruit instead.

✳ Try an activity holiday for a change, and opt for B&B rather than full board so that you won't feel pressured to eat all those 'free' meals.

THE WAY FORWARD

✳

I am still convinced, after hearing from experts all over the world, that fat is not our fault, but it is very much our problem.

While making a TV documentary for Sky Television about real people trying to change their lifestyles in a world that seems to preach 'eat more and exercise less', I witnessed a counselling session between dietitian Lyndel Costain and a young couple, David and Nicola, who were both desperate to lose weight. Lyndel told me that nowadays her advice is less and less about 'what foods are healthy and which foods are not', and more about food behaviour.

'Most people, particularly long-term dieters, know all there is to know about calories and nutritional value,' she told me. 'They know what they should be eating, but they just can't stick to it. That's because it is so very hard to do the opposite of what all the adverts are telling you. From the slimmer's perspective, society is telling you one way to behave, but expecting you to do something else. I tell my clients that they have to kick the diet mentality and get into a totally new mindset – one that is actually at odds with our culture. They have to create their own micro-climate, learn new habits and take small but important steps to change their lifestyle. But it's not easy. The dieting industry, with its unrealistic promises, has set many people up for failure again and again.'

Reaching for the stars

There is absolutely no doubt that the slimming industry sells us products that make questionable claims, but, more harmfully, it encourages us to have unrealistic expectations – just as, over many years, we have been conditioned to aspire to unrealistic body images invented or at least sustained by the media. Dr Gary Foster, director for the Centre for Obesity Research and Education in Philadelphia, says these impractical and improbable goals are one of the main reasons that many patients fail to lose weight at all. Setting yourself too hard a goal actually depresses and demotivates you because the chances are that you'll fall at the first hurdle and then give up. The trouble is, many of the experts I have spoken to suggest that the lower your self-esteem, the higher the goals you set yourself because you so badly need to dream. That's the ultimate cruelty, isn't it? The more you need to lose weight, the more likely you are to suffer from low self-esteem, and the more likely you are to set yourself up for failure and a consequent cycle of making strong resolutions and then 'letting yourself down'. Gary Foster has seen it happen time and again:

'In one study we asked 60 obese women to set themselves four different kinds of goal,' he told me. 'Number one was their "dream weight" – how they saw themselves in their daydreams. Number two was what we called "happy weight" – a size at which they'd feel content. Number three was "acceptable weight" – where they would feel that they had made a discernible achievement and could pat themselves on the back. Finally, number four was their "disappointed weight" – some weight loss, but falling so far short of their hopes that they would feel pretty frustrated. Then they took part in a 48-week weight-loss programme under our supervision. Almost half didn't achieve even their "disappointed weight". Looking back, they realised they had established goals that were way beyond reason.'

But Dr Foster was keen to add that most of the women did indeed lose some fat. 'They saw it as a disappointment, but a loss of just 4 kilos represents a health enhancement in an obese person. That alone can reduce your risk of heart disease, cancer or diabetes... it's significant.'

I have been through this cycle myself – oh, so many times! – and I've now come to one conclusion: if our goals could be more health related than weight related, couldn't a 'disappointing' result be measured for what it really is – one big step in the right direction, or even a 'complete' risk reduction?

Unhelpful fat vocabulary

The words we use to describe just about everything relating to overweight, or weight loss, are so negative. Just look at the following examples from a single day – 2 July 2008 – in the *Daily Mail*. Notice how the same phrase keeps popping up...

> '"I'm sick of being thin," says Natalie Cassidy as she gives up dieting and piles on the pounds... Just three months after being pictured on the beach looking slim and toned, Natalie Cassidy has piled on the pounds again. Natalie, here in London two weeks ago, has decided to abandon her battle with the bulge.'

And then, a couple of pages further inside:

> 'Packing a paunch: disgraced love-rat Darren Day reveals his expanding girth! The former West End star cut a rather podgy figure... His puffy, bloated face rendered him almost unrecognisable... Piling on the pounds: a life of excess appears to have caught up with Darren.'

And as if that wasn't enough:

'Rachel Hunter piles on the pounds...and bursts out of her corset.'

'Piling on the pounds'. I so hate that phrase. For the record, these celebrities were not fat – except perhaps by insane model agency standards. OK, so the Rachel Hunter pictures probably weren't her favourite, but heck, she was appearing in a US television programme called *Celebrity Circus* in which she was showing off her athletic prowess, and yes, she definitely looked more muscly. But to say she had 'piled on the pounds' was plain ridiculous.

'Piling on the pounds' implies, quite disgracefully, that you have deliberately made yourself fat, you've ladled it on, you've spread fat all over yourself in an act of flagrant negligence and stupidity. In fact, in every phrase, headline and picture caption above there's a moral judgement implying wilful self-infliction. Fat people don't develop a disorder, suffer illness or emotional distress, or even undergo a setback (all medically recognised causes of weight gain). They go to a big mountain of fat, get out a spade and shovel it on to themselves. Sinfully and deliberately. What nonsense!

Interestingly, a story about former *EastEnders* actress Natalie Cassidy in *Now* magazine reported her as saying that maintaining her weight loss (she'd dieted from a size 16 to an 8 for a DVD) was simply too stressful. I'm rather glad she said it out loud because so many yo-yo dieters complain privately that they can keep up a stressful, restrictive or strict regime for a short time and lose some weight, but they inevitably revert to their 'old ways', their preferred lifestyle. Natalie said she'd regained a stone and a half, but only the scales would have known. Quite rightly, she protested about having to talk about her weight at all.

'What do I have to do – wear a bikini or Spandex every day just to prove that I haven't put on weight? I'm a bit bored of it all now.'

And 'a source' said: 'She's been enjoying life more and the weight crept back on.' Yes, that's what weight does! It creeps up on us. I haven't yet met a fattie who decided on obesity as a lifestyle choice, yet that is the way the media, many doctors and even a few politicians regard it. However, readers are way ahead of the newspapers themselves, and already questioning media values on the whole subject of fat and obesity, diets and disorders. Their response on the *Daily Mail* website to the stories quoted above demonstrated an entirely different set of values. Overwhelmingly, they blogged that size zero women were unattractive, and that celebrities like Natalie Cassidy looked better with a few more curves. That life was too short to waste time obsessing about a few extra inches here and there. That ordinary people did not want to look like stick insects.

About Natalie Cassidy:

'It's about time we as a society started idolising athletes rather than film stars – that way people would aim to be fitter and healthier, regardless of their physical proportions – that would lead to people being healthily slim, rather than stick thin. It would be a better world if people aimed to be fit, rather than thin. Nearly everyone can achieve a good level of fitness, even if they remain nicely curvy.'
– James, Wigan

And of Rachel Hunter:

'Leave her alone! She looks normal! She looks gorgeous! No wonder so many women are anorexic these days!'
– Vicki, Derby

The print media's spiteful and distorted take on body shape has to stop. It's creating a society in which it's acceptable to disparage anyone who has a less than perfect body, and it's scaring a whole generation of children and young adults into eating disorders.

Television can be just as bad. Last year, after the news broke about Fern Britton's gastric band, I was asked to host a special report on gastric surgery for *The One Show* on the BBC. I agreed to do it provided it wasn't a sensationalised report, and that it was sympathetic to Fern. It was especially important, I knew, to be careful about the words used. I wanted to show that gastric bands aren't a simple, quick-fix solution because they don't work for everyone. So I interviewed one woman who had successfully lost a great deal of weight with hers, and another woman who had lost and then regained weight, despite having a band fitted. 'The winner and the sinner' was the phrase that kept popping up in my research notes from the BBC producers, and I voiced my dislike of that.

'Well, what shall we call them then?' I was asked. 'The winner and the loser? 'Sad and bad? Glad and sad? Sin to win?' (I don't know why, but BBC producers, especially on daytime television, think they're writing a musical comedy. Everything has to be a one-liner, a silly rhyme or a dreadful pun, doesn't it?)

'How about just calling them "people"?' I said.

No one was trying to be unkind, but it was hard work ensuring that we didn't make judgements in every utterance, such as 'doing well' or 'cheating the diet' or 'resorting to desperate measures'. If only we could 'talk up' the whole process of weight loss and slimming. Use better words. Take out the moral judgements. If only we could learn to value health instead of shape and weight, we could adopt better attitudes and respect real values. We might even change the minds of national newspaper editors...

Positive attitude

Minds need changing even within the medical establishment. Strange as it may seem, doctors and other medical professionals actually look down upon obesity specialists, as though that branch of the business is somehow less deserving – less sympathetic. Many surgeons and nurses in bariatrics have told me how they are sneered at by colleagues with other specialisms. Yet obesity specialists are, by and large, a positive lot. That's because, at the moment, they have possibly the only effective 'cure' for obesity.

Diets and lifestyle changes work for some, but surgery often provides the only long-term effective answer for those who have been defeated by other methods. As I've already pointed out, surgery doesn't always work for everyone, and in rare cases it is beginning to show adverse side effects (such as addiction transfer, see page 208), but surgeons tend to see things statistically. Nine times out of 10 their patients report near-miraculous transformations. Add to that the fact that bariatric surgery is a growth industry, so they're constantly in demand, and you can see why they're happy. In the private sector, business is booming.

However – a word of warning: private surgery is largely unregulated. My own experiences show the dangers of what can occur. Aftercare in particular is variable – sometimes barely existent. Some medical companies are so keen to hard sell the band that patients feel pressurised into signing a contract that commits them to a large bill and little information.

NHS – not so healthy

I've become aware that there are people in the medical profession who are not judgemental about the overweight. In fact, they get a real buzz out of helping people so fundamentally regain their quality of life. Could that be because a surprising number of them have weight problems themselves?

This thought came to me when I noticed that a very high proportion of BuddyPower members are nurses, so I asked them why. Why, since nurses are clearly hard-working, intelligent and well informed, do so many of them have a weight problem? Their answers came fast and furious as they complained about long, exhausting shifts and sheer lack of time.

'I come off work absolutely asleep on my feet,' wrote one. 'Then I have a one-hour journey home. The very thought of shopping for healthy food and cooking a healthy meal from raw ingredients when I get home – well, it's just unrealistic! And when could I possibly get to the gym, even if I had the energy? I get so dispirited by the whole thing – and the fact that it's probably only eight hours until my next shift – well, I end up taking the easy option...'

And that is? Buying a couple of Happy Meals on the way home, she said. Which really is convenient, as there's a McDonald's actually in the hospital lobby. Indeed, a high proportion of NHS hospitals have a fast-food franchise right on the premises, licensed to help the hospital make money.

I noticed a similar dearth of healthy options when I took my 'Get Your Life Back' tour to three of Britain's biggest cities at the beginning of 2008. While travelling around, I found myself gasping for a juice bar and a healthy meal. Caffeine and high-calorie fast food were dead easy to come by, but what about my juice? It convinced me, even more than ever, that we're living in a culture that's making us all ill and fat. There I was, stuck in the middle of Birmingham, dehydrating in a hotel room that wouldn't let me turn off the air conditioning, with only instant coffee, UHT milk and a white, processed cheese sandwich on offer. Desperate for something healthy, I asked for a fruit smoothie and was given some glutinous substance in a portion-controlled carton with a straw glued to the side. I walked miles to find a juice bar. In Manchester and Leeds I never found one! I was incensed. No wonder we have an obesity epidemic, with over half the population (that's 20 million adults and a million kids) in danger of losing their health, their childhood or both.

Never mind global warming: we humans won't be around to suffer it – we'll have made ourselves extinct long before the melting ice caps are a problem. We are living in a toxic environment where it's almost impossible to live a healthy life. Obesity isn't just about personal responsibility – it's about the government facing up to theirs. Big time.

After my tour finished, I felt tired, dehydrated, my skin was blotchy, I had baggy eyes and generally felt low, yet the people I'd met and the things we'd discussed had been inspirational. I felt unhealthy because I'd been stressed, drank too much coffee, grabbed junk food because that's all that was available on trains and from room service, and hadn't eaten a proper, balanced meal in days.

Our kids live like that most days. Many skip breakfast, are served up junk at school, and resort to snacking from vending machines and the corner shop. Our nurses and doctors live in a similar world inside the very places that are designed to heal and help us. So let's be brave...

Get rid of junk food outlets from our hospitals and replace them with franchises that promote fruit, juices and quick food that's fresh, nutritious and brimming with the values of a society we want, not one that we're inheriting from the worst of America.

Outlaw all vending machines. Pay off the contracts – it cannot be more expensive than a sick nation that will bankrupt the NHS in 10 years' time if nothing's done.

If the principle of 'you are what you eat' doesn't exist in our hospitals, how can society hope to flourish?

Science versus politics

The doctors and scientists have been warning for years now. They want politicians to see sense and bring in legislation that will require sane, sensible, joined-up thinking. And where better to start than inside the National Health Service? Professor Jimmy Bell, at Imperial College and Hammersmith Hospital in London, agrees, and is angry about the current state of affairs:

'You cannot expect people to work hard for nine or 10 hours a day, spend an hour or two travelling and then go to the gym when they get home. It has to be part of their working life. We have to make it easier to live a healthy lifestyle – and that requires political will and investment. I tell you what – let's get really controversial and radical. Let's stop investing in Trident and invest in our children instead!'

He agrees with Desmond Morris that the human body has evolved to maximise its intake of food, that human beings are animals built for famine and feast, not feast alone. What's more, he says, the evidence suggests that once your body gets fat, it defaults to that position and then fights all attempts to make it lose weight. In other words, your body 'thinks' that obese is the norm and that anything less is wrong. That is why it resists you in your attempts to lose weight.

'As yet, the science behind the theory is pretty weak, but we know it seems to be true – that's why dieting doesn't work very well. Dieting works at first, but then your body shifts back. It makes you crave high sugar and fat to quickly restore your body to its new norm,' he tells me. 'We don't yet know, but suspect that if the mindset is changed early on – in childhood – then it may become almost impossible to reset it.'

Professor Bell describes obesity as a life sentence: 'People liken it to alcoholism, or even an addiction to cigarettes. But it isn't like that. Food is a drug that we all need to exist. The obese person has to learn to limit his addiction – something we ask no other addict to do. You wouldn't tell an alcoholic to learn how to drink just one drink a day. You wouldn't take a cocaine addict to live with a family of drug users and pushers. Yet we tell the food addict, or obese person, to live moderately in an environment packed with food and food advertising. That is why it is so hard for them to beat their problem.

'We scientists have been warning for years how dangerous fat foods are, how we are all getting fatter, but no one listens because of vested interests. The scientists are now coming up with the absolute conclusive proof that people get hooked on fat, sugar and salt, and crave more. But the food industry has known this all along without having to have the scientific proof, and that's why they have put so much sugar, fat and salt in our foods. They could use healthier fats, less sugar and salt if there was a political will. But no one is making them!

'Obesity is a political problem. Yet here we are, looking towards the London Olympics in 2012, and still our government is not addressing our obesogenic environment. They give a very good impression of being worried only about buildings and infrastructure. There is so much more that our culture could do to embrace the real health message behind the Olympics. We might end up the fattest country ever to stage the Games because we are not doing enough already.'

Is there a giant conspiracy afoot? Many scientists and surgeons I have spoken to reckon that political failure to tackle obesity arises from fear: it is just too huge a problem to solve. Politicians would rather see our country go the way of the USA, where health care is privatised, and obesity and its related problems are tackled only by the very rich, who can afford extortionate health premiums.

'It will force a distinction between rich and poor,' explains Professor Bell. 'It is happening in America, and it has already happened in my homeland of Chile. There you have two societies – one rich and able to solve their health problems, and a poor, fat underclass who cannot afford to treat obesity and all its related health conditions.'

Is obesity a class issue?

Already there are signs that obesity is worst in the poorer parts of Britain. There is, as the academics put it, a strong socio-economic divide. Just look at the 'Fat Map' produced last summer as part of the government's National Obesity Strategy. The worst areas – in the northeast, the Midlands and Wales – show that the poorer former industrial and mining towns dominate the 10 fattest areas, while the affluent people from wealthier areas in London and the Home Counties dominate the 10 slimmest. In fact, Camden in north London, where I lived for many years, was one of the slimmest areas in the whole country. When I think back, I remember it was 'fashionable', full of trendy sushi restaurants and positively bulging with health clubs and gyms. If I still lived there, perhaps my famous battle with the bulge would have been enough to skew the figures and knock it off the 'healthiest' pedestal!

We certainly saw an example of the class divide recently on TV, where a former member of our royal family sought to change the eating habits of a working-class family on a council estate in Humberside. *The Duchess in Hull* showed Fergie – Sarah, Duchess of York – take her own healthy eating message into a kitchen where microwave meals and Pot Noodles were the norm – and the family was fat and keen to change their ways. The newspapers responded with derision. But I found Fergie articulate and well informed on the problems facing perhaps not so many of *her* class, but a whole generation of TV viewers.

In the USA Sarah is an ambassador for WeightWatchers. Even now she has shed her excess weight and is slim and nimble, she says she couldn't maintain her new weight without the constant help of the WW experts.

'In fact, when they first approached me, I thought I could become their ambassador just by talking the talk,' she confided in me. 'I thought I could just carry on with the lifestyle I was leading – with my weight going up and down all the time. But they insisted I do the programme. Of course, now I am glad they did because it taught me a lot. And I couldn't stay slim now without their help.'

Sarah puts her weight problem down to the feelings of loss and abandonment she experienced when her mother famously left home to go and live with an Argentinian polo player, half a world away, when she was just 12. Until then, Sarah had been living the dream life of a little girl born to wealthy parents – the sort of family who could indulge her childish wish to have her very own gymkhana.

'It was wonderful. We even had our own rosettes with the name of the farm, and there were sweets for all the winners,' she remembers. But shortly after the gymkhana, her mother left home. Sarah remembers going to the room where the sweets were stored.

'There were loads left over. They were Opal Fruits – I remember them so well! And I sat and ate them to comfort myself. From that moment, sugar became my friend.'

Other people, she reckons, need to look at their own personal reasons for comfort eating. Some might have a weight problem caused by a chemical imbalance or something missing in their lives; with other people it could be a form of depression.

'Not with me,' she said. 'In my case it was due to a feeling of great loss [about] my mother... I turned to food as my comfort to numb the hole in my heart. I definitely, definitely know that I eat to compensate for feelings. I am sure it's an addiction. It's the easiest form of "drug". Drinking, smoking, taking drugs are all no-nos, but food is so readily available and you can do it very quietly and so easily hide your overeating – it's a way of pampering yourself.'

Now Sarah campaigns in the United States, where she has joined the list of celebrities endorsing the major weight-reduction companies. She hopes one day to be taken seriously in the UK, but until then, she spreads the word however she can: 'I tell everyone...my five points, my tips. If I can help just one person, then I feel it's been worthwhile.'

1   Watch your water intake. Anyone can go to the tap – it's free and easy, and it's important.

2   Take tiny baby steps to weight loss – don't think you are going to lose 5 lb in a weekend.

3   Exercise – there's no question that it's important. Try running upstairs. One of my best friends said to me. 'Remember, Fergie,

any steps are to be run, never walked, wherever you are, and never, never take the elevator!'

4   Try to learn what foods are good for you and your body. Listen to your body – it will tell you. If something gives you indigestion, don't eat it, try something else, it just isn't suitable for you. Don't make food bland – always take some balsamic vinegar with you or something to add a little flavour.

5   Love yourself. Self-esteem is very important. Realise you are doing your best, you are only human, you're doing OK!

It might sound like simple advice, but until the scientists come up with the ultimate slimming pill – one that curbs your appetite, makes you feel fuller sooner and has no side effects – it's almost all there is.

The magic bullet

Professor Jane Wardle, at University College Hospital, London, looks forward to the day when fat people will be prescribed anti-obesity pills without any moral judgement – just as people with high blood pressure are prescribed medication.

'Actually, it wasn't many years ago that moral judgements *were* made about people who had high blood pressure because we knew that much of the condition was caused by carrying too much weight, or eating a "bad" diet, rich in fatty foods. If you had high blood pressure, all your doctor could tell you to do was go away, lose weight, do some exercise, avoid alcohol and reduce the salt in your food. More often than not, you couldn't reverse your condition because, well, those things are hard, so hard, to do. In fact, the moral judgements only stopped when the drugs were invented. Suddenly doctors, patients and the outside world started to recognise that high blood pressure was a serious condition, and not just a cue for holier-than-thou opinions.

'The advent of an effective medicine actually brought about new thinking and stopped a great deal of prejudice. Perhaps the same will happen to obesity, and then the lucky ones who don't suffer from weight problems will start to think of it as more of a medical condition than a self-inflicted state of sin. Scientists are working on it right now. The race is on to find the world's first no-risk drug, free of side effects, which would help people lose fat and then control their weight. There's big, big money in whoever makes it first.

'Let's be plain. I'm not talking about a gluttony drug – one that will allow you to eat whatever you want and damn the consequences. What's needed is a drug that will help your body to eat like a slim person – in moderation, without the bewildering craving for more – and that will ensure your body won't go into famine mode, turning every little calorie into fat to store for future lean times. You know...something like today's adverts promise, but fail to deliver.'

In other words, a drug that will balance out your 'fat genes'. Jane wishes she had it – and soon – because she knows it would transform lives.

'I think one day we may find something that really helps. We mustn't be Luddite and say we can't do such things to the body because we *already are* doing that. We have to try and see this as a balance. Look at the daily medications that do give people their life back – everything from statins to pain control drugs. You cannot deny their effectiveness. People want to get on with their life, and if we can help them do that, surely that is a good thing to do?

'And then there's the fact that taking a daily drug often concentrates the mind and makes patients more determined to help themselves too. Sometimes the advent of effective medical treatments actually makes people sit up and take notice of their own problem a bit more than before. People might say, "Actually, I don't want to take this drug for the rest of my life. Perhaps cutting down on my food intake, changing my lifestyle, doing more exercise, perhaps that's not such a bad price to pay after all." Until that drug comes along, though, the fight against flab is painfully tortuous.'

However, I can tell you that a 'magic bullet' is surprisingly close. In fact, they have already started phase one of human trials. And what exactly is it? Well, it's an injection of a substance derived from a hormone that we all naturally produce in the gut. It tells the brain when the stomach has had enough. It gives you a feeling of satiety. In fact, when word of it first got out and it was mooted that it could even be put into certain foodstuffs, say chewing gum, it gave rise to the headline:

'The Gum That Slims Your Bum!'

Professor Steve Bloom, who's based at Hammersmith Hospital and is the chief of all the pioneering fat work being undertaken, is particularly amused by that headline, but says it's all nonsense.

'It's never going to be put into a chewing gum, but we have got it into a form that is injectable. One day, it could be available, for instance, in a reusable syringe pen, and that might be a very useful alternative for patients who need a gastric bypass.'

He explained: 'It's a hormone that tells the brain: "Stop the supply because we'll explode!" Evolution has made us reasonably efficient [at controlling food intake] by giving us a control system that temporarily switches off hunger after we've had a meal, or when the gut isn't well and cannot cope. That's the hormone we've managed to isolate and reproduce. Bariatric surgeons know that this is the substance that comes into play particularly efficiently for patients who have had a gastric bypass: they hardly ever feel hungry, and are completely satisfied after only a very little food.

'Bypass surgery is potentially dangerous. It's also very expensive, and we don't even know that it always works, although the evidence is good. I would like to do the same thing medically for people with a big weight problem as is achieved surgically – jabs instead of surgery.'

All it needs is half a billion quid, he says. But, even with drugs companies champing at the bit for the right formula, that's difficult money to raise. At the moment, with £10 million stumped up, they're at the stage called 'phase one human trials'. This means the drug has been given to about 60 people. Now the long process of evaluation must take place before the next stage, and the next and so on. So even at conservative estimates, it couldn't possibly be on the market for another 10 years, and who knows what hurdles might have to be overcome in that time? By then, more than half the world could be obese.

Does Professor Bloom think it ethical to live in a world where more than half the population could be injecting themselves every day just to stay slim? Isn't that – to use the terrible tabloid term – cheating?

'Ah, well,' he responds dryly, 'I think when you go to the States you ought to swim because it is clearly cheating to go on a plane. And you ought to have your own orchestra at home when you want to listen to music because listening via an iPod is cheating... There's no point in being an oughtist.'

An oughtist?

'Too many people are oughtists. They talk of what we ought to do... [But] we aren't always in control of ourselves – certain needs are built into us. We are a famine-surviving species. We are the top of an evolutionary tree where eating is essential...

'I am not suggesting half the world takes an injection every day. Nutritionists and dietary clinicians are trying to approach the problem in a different way, and the two approaches should be able to dovetail.'

The professor points out that in a future world that has overcome famine, where delicious, high-calorie foods are heavily advertised, where people ride rather than walk, there will be an obesity pandemic because we are ill adapted to that environment. 'In that case we have to do something artificial to compensate. For example, if you live in Greenland, where it is very cold, you need extra warm clothing, otherwise you would freeze to death... That is entirely artificial [but] you have to do it to overcome a hostile environment, and nobody feels that's unnatural or wrong.

'So we have this new [obesogenic] environment to which we are not adapted, with plentiful food and no need for exercise. We must take action to adapt. Either you have lots of self-control, which has been shown to be an utter failure, or you have to change the food, the advertising...or force people to exercise every day... but you cannot just say people ought to be all right because clearly they aren't... The logic is that if you accept the changes in our environment, then you must accept the consequences.'

And that could be a daily injection to fight the flab. Morally wrong or just plain practical? Would this be society abdicating all blame, or the ultimate acceptance of liability?

What next?

Sadly, it seems that tomorrow's politicians (or, at least, those who aspire to being tomorrow's government) want to shirk any liability for obesity. They want fatties told, as they enter the doctor's door, that they are obese because they eat too much and exercise too little. In fact, Tory leader David Cameron actually gave a speech in Glasgow in July 2008 in which he said he was fed up of hearing that people were 'at risk of obesity', and accused anyone suffering from obesity, or alcoholism or drug addiction, of 'moral neutrality', against which he would henceforth speak out! Thanks to his high profile, the headlines reporting his speech were all rather scornful, along the lines of 'Fatties have only themselves to blame'. Alan Johnson, Labour's health minister, said 'permission to be cruel and nasty about the obese has now been granted by the leader of the opposition'.

At least the minister has woken up to the scale of the problem, and warned in no uncertain terms of its dangers to society as a whole. Like the Americans, he has used dramatic language, such as 'the biggest health threat facing us', but he seems to understand the downright humanity of the issue. In a recent speech he said: 'Just as the government has a moral duty to tackle poverty and exclusion, so it also has a duty to address obesity. But this is not a licence to hector and lecture people on how they should spend their lives – not least because that approach simply won't work. Tackling obesity requires a much broader partnership, not only with families, but with employers, retailers, the leisure industry, the media, local government and the voluntary sector. We need a national movement that will bring about a fundamental change in the way we live our lives.'

Hear, hear! If we have a change in government quite soon, can we keep Alan Johnson, please? He's talking the only sort of language that can deliver change.

It is important that society understands why fat is such a big problem. It needs expert solutions – from behavioural therapists right through to the big drugs companies. I am thrilled that at last government is taking it seriously, with its Change4Life initiatives, promoting fitness and healthy eating. I applaud the move to get the food industry and fast food companies on board, though I doubt they'll ever do anything that'll compromise profits. Putting 'I'm a thriller in the griller' on a packet of bacon won't, I predict, make Mum shun a fry-up, nor will voluntary measures be enough to ensure a lifestyle revolution.

Obesity is happening right across the world – in startling numbers and to kids of every colour, race and creed. It's in Japan, China and India, and now Australia is officially the most obese nation on Earth. Does David Cameron think that all of humanity has suddenly lost its sense of personal responsibility? Yes, some of us are greedy pigs and lazy too, but not most of us. Yes, some of us have become indolent and benefit-dependent, blaming others for our corpulent guts and thin wallets. But not all of us. Yes, some of us are couch potatoes and Internet addicts, who shy away from the sunlight and groan at the thought of crossing the road to buy another can of beer. But definitely not all of us.

The reason so much of the world's population is now 'at risk of obesity' is because our culture, our Western lifestyle, is conducive to obesity, heart disease, diabetes, stroke and cancer. Highly processed and nutrient-poor foods are cheaper than fresh fruits, vegetables and meats; and who's been taught to cook anyway? Sedentary living, the prevalence of processed, junk food, an instinctive lack of faith in our environment – dangerous roads, dark pavements and street crime – all contribute. As a nation, we're scared of letting our kids play outside: it's easier and safer, we think, to let them play on the computer.

Of course obesity is a matter of personal responsibility, but it is also society's responsibility to make the environment healthier. Society *can* be changed. It has happened in Finland, where in 20 years they have gone from fat-loving, heart-attack victims to exercise-mad, healthy eaters. Their obesity rate was twice *then* what ours is us *now*. They had the highest rate of heart attacks in Europe. Now their lifestyle has become the envy of the world. How did they do it? Shouldn't our politicians be asking that question? The doctor who made the difference in Finland says: 'Healthy choices need to be easy choices, and when they are, people make them.'

We haven't time to moralise; we need to get on with a plan that works. An acceptance of personal responsibility has to be one factor, but so does social responsibility, and that comes from our political leaders. They need to make the changes that will help us all to help ourselves. That is a true marriage of social and personal responsibility.

Individually we must not shirk our share of the blame. We all know, don't we, that we are eating too much and moving too little? As parents too, we owe it to our kids to put our own house in order. But we have to be helped by a caring society that, if not being our nanny, can at least be a caring aunt or uncle.

At the start of my quest for an answer to the problem of obesity, I spent an afternoon with a man who used to be Tony Blair's senior policy adviser on health. He's Julian Le Grand, professor of social policy at the London School of Economics. He was the man who once suggested that there was nothing wrong with a nanny state because we needed it. He suggested we change the default in society, where the healthy option becomes the state-enforced norm, so that we have the freedom to opt out. On smoking, for instance, he said, what about a blanket ban – everywhere? But if you wanted to smoke, you could: you would just need to apply for a licence to smoke in certain areas. Similarly, he reckoned we should stop the escalators and lifts from working (except for the disabled) below the second floor in any high-rise building, and that companies should provide 'exercise hours' for their workforce, which everyone would be expected to take part in unless they deliberately chose not to. He also advocated a total ban on salt in processed foods. This would hand control of salt content to the consumer, who could choose to 'opt out' of the healthy product by adding salt at the table.

I listened to him talk about his ideas for what he calls 'libertarian paternalism', where the state tries to make healthy decisions for you, and I thought: 'Perhaps this sort of nannying is OK because it treats everyone the same – provides a healthy level playing field for all,' as opposed to the Ealing initiative that targeted just smokers [see page 102]. What's wrong with embracing a healthier society – or should we go on, blindly defending our right to kill ourselves in the name of freedom of choice? In matters of health, which impacts on the ability of the National Health Service to provide welfare, surely such nannying is a good thing? I liked his idea that supermarkets could be required to sell alcohol separately from groceries, thus requiring customers to queue twice, or that the sale of alcohol could be restricted to off-licences (as used to be the case in the United States), requiring an extra journey – and extra effort – by the consumer. Personally, I reckon that making it just that little bit harder to buy cream cakes and peanuts might be helpful too...

That's a good idea! We're all like sheep to a certain extent. We'll follow if someone leads us in the right direction...as a group of university researchers recently discovered. They chose a big department store and put a sign at the foot of both the stairs and the escalators, reading: 'It's much healthier for you if you take the stairs!' and then they filmed the reaction. Surges of shoppers making their way towards the escalators changed their mind and trudged up the steps. The sign clearly tweaked their conscience and they took the healthier option. This continued for several weeks, and still the shoppers took the stairs instead of the escalator – they didn't tire of the message. Then the sign was taken away and immediately everyone reverted to the escalator. A week later, the sign was put back, and again it had the original effect – a return to the stairs.

Yes, we're like sheep! We have the healthy message inside our head, but our body will take the easy option unless constantly reminded. Now advertisers know this, otherwise they'd pay for just one advert to tell us that chocolate is a wonderful luxury we all deserve, or that ready-made meals are incredibly quick and convenient. They know we need telling again and again or we'll forget. So the healthy message needs to be reinforced with the same sort of vigour, and it must be made easy for us to get fit and eat well. At the moment, our problem is gigantic because we've got our fitness and eating habits out of proportion.

I recently met Sian Porter, a leading nutritionist from the Fat Panel, an independent body of obesity experts, who reckons we're all shockingly ignorant about saturated fats and how to avoid them. (In fact, there's been a lot of shocking news about obesity. Did you see the report that half of all British women cannot do up their own bra?) Sian Porter says we should be taught 'easy to remember' guidelines for portion sizes, the absolute key to getting us back on track. And the 'buy one get one free' culture is, she says, one of the biggest evils in the fight against fat. If you think it's a bargain, you should ask at what price to your health.

I reckon that every advertising break on the TV should include quickie little reminders like these:

* If it's not in the house, you can't eat it
* Keep the fruit bowl full and the biscuit tin empty.
* If you want a biscuit, put it off for 20 minutes, as the craving often goes away.

✳ Always have a piece of fruit in your bag or desk or car.

✳ Go for a parking space far from the car park exit.

✳ If you are going to have something alcoholic, drink some water first to slake your thirst.

✳ Always have a jug of water at the meal table.

✳ Eat more fish.

Meanwhile, I've just started wearing a pedometer (again). You know how we are all meant to do at least 10,000 steps a day? Well, one day recently I got up early to cook breakfast for the kids and took them to school. Then I dashed down the motorway to Heathrow Airport and caught an early flight to Belfast. I did five interviews with the Irish media and then spoke at a lunch for Breast Cancer Care. I then went to a TV studio and did another interview, then caught the afternoon flight back, and arrived in time to go and see my youngest son in a school concert. When I got home that evening, I helped with the homework, did my emails and then fell into bed, utterly exhausted. The pedometer told me that I'd done 813 steps – yes, that's right – eight hundred and thirteen.

That's what I mean by a sedentary lifestyle. It's certainly not a lazy one, but that's why I'm still fighting the flab. Energy in is not equalling energy out. Which is why I recommend this little gadget on my waistband. Like Jiminy Cricket, it's my conscience, but not as loveable.

Meanwhile, as the debate continues, I am sure of one thing: the power of health campaigning. I learnt the lesson with the 'Back to Sleep' campaign (see page 48), still the UK's most successful health campaign ever. While the politicians told me that it was enough to tell young mothers in hospital the new advice that babies should sleep on their back, I demanded a TV advertising campaign. I said we needed the adverts to be short, sharp, easy to understand, and they should air on morning TV and in the *Coronation Street* advertising breaks. Later it was found that some 80 per cent of mothers who were aware of the new Back to Sleep advice had got it from television.

Now we need another TV campaign because obesity is killing not only mums and dads, but children too.

Remember my shocking fact about childhood obesity causing type 2 diabetes, which in turn poses a very high risk of making our children impotent or infertile? That fact alone should be the basis of a campaign. In Australia it caused a virtual stampede of interest from anxious mums demanding to know how to safeguard their children's future and their own right to have grandchildren! Well, every night a hard-hitting TV ad should be reminding us that our lifestyle is killing us and wrecking our kids' future. Backed up behind it should be a raft of social and environmental initiatives to help us change. Why are we pussyfooting around on this issue? Have we learnt nothing from the smoking saga? Have we learnt nothing from the advertising industry? There's a reason they spend millions on extravagant filming and catchy slogans: people remember the message, and they respond.

If we spent as much money on advertising grapes and apples as is spent on Mars bars and Pot Noodles, would we see a revolution? Could the celery stick become the must-have, iconic ingredient in our kids' lunch-boxes? Could sporting superheroes such as David Beckham inspire a new generation with superlative adverts for broccoli instead of Brylcreem? Courgettes instead of cola? Mushrooms instead of mobile phones?

I really don't know. Perhaps no one does. But to me it seems immoral not to try.

BIBLIOGRAPHY AND REFERENCES

*

While every effort has been made to acknowledge all copyright holders, the publisher apologises for any errors and invites readers to notify them of any omissions.

My Story

McCaffrey, J. and Hoyle, A. (2006), 'Anne Diamond stomach op killed my girl' in the *Daily Mirror*, 7 February 2006

NICE – National Institute for Clinical Excellence (2006), *Obesity: Guidance on the prevention, identification, assessment and management of overweight and obesity in adults and children*, NICE clinical guideline 43, December 2006, page 11

Chapter 1 – Fat Is a Four-letter Word

BBC (2007), *Mary Queen of Shops*, TV series

Carlin, George (2006), *Brain Droppings*, Hyperion

Crewe, Candida (2006), *Eating Myself*, Bloomsbury

Dempsey, Karen (2007), 'Government comes under pressure to make discrimination against obese people illegal', *Personnel Today*, 13 March 2007

Diamond, Anne (2007), 'Anyone who's fat or obese is used to life being unfair', *Personnel Today*, 12 March 2007

Frith, Maxine (2003), 'Scientist's claim on cot death is flawed, Appeal Court hears', the *Independent*, 5 December 2003

Golding, William (1954), *Lord of the Flies*, Faber

Higgins, Charlotte (2006), 'The fat lady slims', the *Guardian*, 26 September 2006

Lampert, Leslie (1993), 'Fat like me', *Ladies' Home Journal*, May 1993

Management in Practice (2007), 'Fat people face prejudice in the workplace, says survey', *Management in Practice*, 12 March 2007

McGibbon, Rob (2006), 'The press conference with Peter Stringfellow', pressgazette.co.uk, 10 February 2006 (http://www.robmcgibbon.com/resources/pcw_peter_stringfellow.pdf)

Moore, Judith (2005), *Fat Girl*, Profile Books

Nolan, Stephen (2008), 'Too fat to drive a bus?' (www.bbc.co.uk/northernireland/nolan/catchuptv/69.shtml)

Park, Justin,H., et al., 'Pathogen-avoidance mechanisms and the stigmatization of obese people' *Evolution and Human Behaviour*, Volume 28, Issue 6, pages 410–14, as reported in Fernandez, Colin, 'Scientists discover why thin people dislike fat people', the *Daily Mail*, 30 July 2007

Paton, Graeme (2007), 'Authors "making fat children bully targets"', the *Daily Telegraph*, 12 May 2007

Personnel Today (2007), 'Fattism in the workplace: reader responses to our "F-word" obesity feature', *Personnel Today*, 3 April 2007

Rowling, J.K. (1997), *Harry Potter and the Philosopher's Stone*, Bloomsbury

Smith, David (2007), 'BBC Dragon: I wouldn't like to hire fat people', the *Observer* 22 April 2007

Webb, Dr Jean (2008), 'Voracious appetites: the construction of "fatness" in children's literature', in Keeling, K. and Pollard, S. (eds.), *Critical Approaches to Food and Children's Literature*, Routledge

Chapter 2 – Appearances Can Be Deceptive

Snyderman, Nancy (2007), *Living Large in America: Inside the Body*, TV documentary, NBC 27 October 2007

Wake up, Whitehall!

All Party Parliamentary Group on Obesity (2004), 'Report on Obesity', 27 May 2004

NICE – National Institute for Clinical Excellence (2006), *Obesity: Guidance on the prevention, identification, assessment and management of overweight and obesity in adults and children*, NICE clinical guideline 43, December 2006, page 11

Norwich Union Healthcare (2003–present), 'Health of the Nation', ongoing research programme (www.healthofthenation.com)

Social Justice Policy Group (2006), 'Breakdown Britain: Interim report on the health of the nation', the Centre for Social Justice

Chapter 3 – Is There Really an Obesity Epidemic?

Basham, Patrick (2006), *Diet Nation: Exposing the Obesity Crusade*, Social Affairs Unit

Basham, Patrick and Luik, John (2008), 'Is the obesity epidemic exaggerated? Yes', *British Medical Journal*, 2 February 2008

Basham, Patrick (forthcoming), *Dying to Diet: A Practitioner's Personal Story*

Feinmann, Jane, 'Obesity "epidemic": Who are you calling fat?', interview with Patrick Basham, the *Independent*, 23 October 2007

Government Office for Science (2007), 'Foresight' report, 'Tackling Obesities: Future Choices – Modelling Future Trends in Obesity and Their Impact on Health', Government Office for Science

Guilano, Mireille (2004), *French Women Don't Get Fat!*, Chatto & Windus

Love, John F. (1995), *McDonald's: Behind the Arches*, Bantam Books, page 423, as quoted in the *Independent*, 26 September 2004

Saberi, Roxana (2005), 'Iranians tackle rise in obesity', *BBC News*, Isfahan, 28 December 2005 (http://news.bbc.co.uk/1/hi/world/middle_east/4563776.stm)

Stewart, Simon, et al. (2008), 'Australia's Future "Fat Bomb"' report, Baker IDI Heart & Diabetes Institute

Why the Naked Ape Has Become Obese

Morris, Desmond (1967), *The Naked Ape*, Jonathan Cape

Morris, Desmond (1977), *Manwatching*, Jonathan Cape

Morris, Desmond (2002), *Peoplewatching*, Vintage

Chapter 4 – The Fat Difference between Men and Women

Prescott, John (2008), *Prezza: My Story*, Headline

Bill Clinton and Childhood Obesity

China Daily (2004), http://www.chinadaily.com.cn/english/doc/2004-09/07/content_372401.htm

Clinton, Bill (2005a), 'We must act now', *Parade Magazine*, 25 September 2005

Clinton, Bill (2005b), *My Life*, Arrow

Clinton, Hillary (2004), http://www.clintonfoundation.org/news/news-media/090604-nr-cf-gn-hrt-st-senator-clinton-on-outcome-of-wjc-heart-bypass-surgery

Gupta, Dr Sanjay (2005a) 'Bill Clinton and weight', TV interview, *House Call*, CNN, 6 August 2005 (http://edition.cnn.com/2005/HEALTH/diet.fitness/08/05/clinton.obesity/index.html)

Gupta, Dr Sanjay (2005b), 'Clinton: "I was a fat band boy"', press release, CNN, 7 August 2005 (http://edition.cnn.com/2005/HEALTH/diet.fitness/08/05/clinton.obesity/index.html)

WHO – World Health Organisation (1997), *Obesity: Preventing and Managing the Global Epidemic*, Report of a WHO Consultation on Obesity, 3–5 June 1997, Geneva, WHO Technical Report Series 984

Chapter 5 – Fat Kids Make Fat Adults

Herbert, Ian (2007), 'Oliver's plan fails as pupils snub school meals', the *Independent*, 4 September 2007

Voices against Child Abusity

Alliance for a Healthier Generation (www.healthiergeneration.org)

Clinton, Bill (2005a), 'We must act now', *Parade Magazine*, 25 September 2005

Government Office for Science (2007), 'Foresight' report, (2007), 'Tackling Obesities: Future Choices – Modelling Future Trends in Obesity and Their Impact on Health', Government Office for Science

Huckabee, Mike (2005), *Quit Digging Your Grave with a Knife and Fork*, Center Street

OGSC – Office of the Governor of the State of California (2007), 'Governor Schwarzenegger and President Clinton join forces to fight childhood obesity', Office of the Governor of the State of California, 19 September 2007 (http://gov.ca.gov/speech/7478)

Squires, Sally (2004), 'The Governor is a Happy Loser', *Washington Post*, 10 August 2004

Chapter 6 – The Psychology of Fat

Smith, Dr Robin, interview on 'Suddenly Skinny', *The Oprah Winfrey Show* (http://www.oprah.com/slideshow/oprahshow/oprahshow1_ss_20061024/8)

The Way Forward

Foster, Dr Gary, et al. (2008), Obesity Map in 'Weighing up the burden of obesity', report sponsored by Roche Products Ltd

INDEX

ACKNOWLEDGEMENTS

I would like to thank the following people for agreeing to be interviewed for the book.

Particular thanks go to Former President of the United States **Bill Clinton** and The Clinton Foundation for permission to reproduce excerpts from speeches included in 'Bill Clinton and childhood obesity' and Chapter 5; **Arnold Schwarzenegger** and the Office of the Governor of the State of California; and **Mike Huckabee** for quotes from speeches included in Chapter 5.

Also to: **Andrew Lansley**, health spokesman for the Conservative Party; **Mr Roger Ackroyd**, consultant general surgeon; **Prof Patrick Basham**, author of *Diet Nation*; **Prof Jimmy Bell**, head of the Molecular Imaging Group at the Medical Research Council; **Prof Stephen R. Bloom**, Imperial College; **Prof Robert Bucholz**, Loyola University, Chicago; **Dr David Bull**, broadcaster and campaigner; **Matt Capehorn**, National Obesity Forum; **Keith and Juliane Davis**; **Jane deVille Almond**, independent nurse consultant; **Louise Diss**, The Obesity Awareness and Solutions Trust (TOAST); **Prof John Dixon**, head of obesity research, Monash University; **Kristina Downing-Orr**, clinical psychologist and broadcaster; **Iain Duncan Smith MP**; **Prof Garry Egger**, creator of Professor Trim's Weight Loss for Men (www.professortrim.com); **Prof Gary D. Foster**,

Center for Obesity Research and Education, Temple University; **Tam Fry**, the Child Growth Foundation; **Francine Hodges**; **Chris Jessop**; **Leslie Lampert**; **Betty McBride**, British Heart Foundation; **Mr Mike McMahon**, Professor of Surgery, University of Leeds; **Dr Anoop Misra**, director and head, Department of Diabetes and Metabolic Diseases, Fortis Group of Hospitals (New Delhi, NOIDA, and Jessaram) and head of the Indian Obesity Task Force; **Desmond Morris**, zoologist, author and artist; **Marie Parker**; **Sian Porter**, dietitian and adviser on the Fat Panel (www.thefatpanel. org.uk); **Prof Carol Propper**, Bristol University; **Dr Asad Rahim**, consultant in obesity and endocrinology; **MeMe Roth**, president and founder of the US group National Action Against Obesity; **Prof Dr Carmen Russoniello**, North Carolina University; **Dr Nizal Sarrafzadegan**, Isfahan Healthy Heart Programme; **Jonathan Scott and family**; **Nancy Snyderman**, chief medical editor for NBC News; **Mr Shaw Somers**, consultant specialist surgeon; **Prof Simon Stewart**, Baker Heart Research Institute; **Prof Boyd Swinburn**, Deakin University; **Dr Colin Waine**, National Obesity Forum; **Prof Jane Wardle**, University of London; **Elspeth Watt**, Calibre HR & Training; **Prof Jean Webb**, International Research Centre: Children's literature, literacy and creativity, University of Worcester; **Carnie Wilson**, American singer and TV host.

A special thank you to **Sarah, Duchess of York**.

And finally, thank you to my agent, Tony Fitzpatrick, my commissioning editor Emma Swaisland, and all who have been willing to share their experiences with others on the BuddyPower website.

The publishers would like to thank Trish Burgess for her editing and Annette Peppis for text design.